Advance praise for
The Sierras Weight-Loss Solution for Teens and Kids

"Any and every health professional who has contact with obese children *must* have this book in their library . . . better even . . . on their desks. Even better still, order dozens of copies and make sure that every parent with an overweight child gets this book and wears out its pages with overuse."

—PETER NEIMAN, M.D., DIRECTOR, PEDIATRIC OBESITY CLINIC OF CALGARY

"Simple, efficient, effective . . . The Sierras Solution's novel weight-loss system has helped young people lose weight when other approaches fail. The emphasis on fresh produce, nonfat dairy, and lean protein provides a lifelong opportunity to maintain health and weight."

—GEORGIA KOSTAS, MPH, R.D., L.D., AUTHOR OF *THE COOPER CLINIC SOLUTION TO THE DIET REVOLUTION* AND FORMER NUTRITION DIRECTOR, COOPER CLINIC, DALLAS

"In my wide range of work with people who suffer from excess weight, I have always looked for a solution such as the one Dr. Kirschenbaum and his colleagues have proposed. When I first heard about the Academy of the Sierras, I quickly recognized their unique approach to working with obese adolescents. Now in this wonderful new book, they again reveal the truth of the science: careful assessment, cognitive behavior therapy, and an emphasis on developing healthy obsessions, including high levels of activity, prove the science true again and again. As important as the science are the heroic stories of these young men and women and the fruits of their work toward conquering their obesity. This book reveals a truly inspiring approach to successful weight loss."

—JOHN RABKIN, M.D., DIRECTOR, PACIFIC LAPAROSCOPY; FORMER ASSOCIATE PROFESSOR OF SURGERY, OREGON HEALTH AND SCIENCES UNIVERSITY

"Finally! A book that can help children and their families succeed. As a health psychologist who has worked with so many desperate families, it is refreshing to find a book that doesn't stop at offering eating and exercising tips. Dr. Kirschenbaum and his colleagues anticipate every "What if . . ." and "Yes, but . . ." question that comes up along the bumpy road to success.

I can't wait to recommend this book to the families with whom I work and my professional colleagues."

—EILEEN ROSENDAHL, PH.D., CLINICAL PSYCHOLOGIST, NEW YORK

"*The Sierras Weight-Loss Solution for Teens and Kids* gets to the heart of the matter. . . . Weight loss is a family affair. This book provides parents with clear, practical advice on how to partner with their child and provide unwavering support and encouragement in their weight-loss journey. The authors state that 'Knowing the enemy is the first step to beating it!' This book shows you how to beat 'it' once and for all and achieve long-term success."

—JUDY E. MARSHEL, PH.D., R.D., CDN, FORMER SENIOR NUTRITIONIST AT WEIGHT WATCHERS INTERNATIONAL, CORPORATE CONSULTANT, AND NUTRITION THERAPIST FOR THE LIVE LIGHT—LIVE RIGHT WEIGHT CONTROL PROGRAM AT BROOKDALE UNIVERSITY HOSPITAL AND MEDICAL CENTER, NEW YORK

"Dr. Kirschenbaum and his colleagues demonstrate in their wonderful new book, *The Sierras Weight-Loss Solution for Teens and Kids,* that it is very possible and remarkably helpful to marry the art and science of medicine, where 'human value' is as cherished as 'statistical value.' Their approach is the genuine article."

—H. VONDELL CLARK, M.D., MPH, MEDICAL DIRECTOR, CATAWBA VALLEY MEDICAL CENTER WEIGHT MANAGEMENT CENTER, NORTH CAROLINA

"Dr. Kirschenbaum is a leading researcher and clinician in the area of childhood obesity. He is committed to helping children lead more healthy lives. The Sierras Weight-Loss Solution and the extension of his work to boarding schools and camps are very innovative approaches to this very difficult pediatric problem."

—NEIL J. HOCHSTADT, PH.D., PROFESSOR OF PEDIATRICS, DEPARTMENT OF PEDIATRICS, THE UNIVERSITY OF CHICAGO, AND DIRECTOR, BEHAVIORAL SCIENCES DEPARTMENT, LA RABIDA CHILDREN'S HOSPITAL, CHICAGO

The Sierras Weight-Loss Solution

for Teens and Kids

Daniel S. Kirschenbaum, Ph.D.,
Ryan Craig, JD,
and Lisa Tjelmeland, MSW

PENGUIN
CANADA

The Sierras Weight-Loss Solution for Teens and Kids

A Scientifically Based Program

from the Highly Acclaimed

Weight-Loss School

PENGUIN CANADA

Published by the Penguin Group

Penguin Group (Canada), 90 Eglinton Avenue East, Suite 700, Toronto, Ontario,
    Canada M4P 2Y3 (a division of Pearson Canada Inc.)

Penguin Group (USA) Inc., 375 Hudson Street, New York, New York 10014, U.S.A.
Penguin Books Ltd, 80 Strand, London WC2R 0RL, England
Penguin Ireland, 25 St Stephen's Green, Dublin 2, Ireland (a division of Penguin Books Ltd)
Penguin Group (Australia), 250 Camberwell Road, Camberwell, Victoria 3124, Australia
    (a division of Pearson Australia Group Pty Ltd)
Penguin Books India Pvt Ltd, 11 Community Centre, Panchsheel Park, New Delhi–110 017, India
Penguin Group (NZ), 67 Apollo Drive, Rosedale, North Shore 0745, Auckland, New Zealand
    (a division of Pearson New Zealand Ltd.)
Penguin Books (South Africa) (Pty) Ltd, 24 Sturdee Avenue, Rosebank, Johannesburg 2196, South Africa

Penguin Books Ltd, Registered Offices: 80 Strand, London WC2R 0RL, England

First published in Canada by Penguin Group (Canada), a division of Pearson Canada Inc., 2007.
Simultaneously published in the United States by Avery, an imprint of Penguin Group U.S.A.

10 9 8 7 6 5 4 3 2 1

Manufactured in the U.S.A.

ISBN-13: 978-0-14-305535-8
ISBN-10: 0-14-305535-6

Book design by Lovedog Studio

Library and Archives of Canada Canadian Cataloguing in Publication data available upon request.
American Library of Congress Cataloging in Publication data available.

Visit the Penguin Group (Canada) website at **www.penguin.ca**

Special and corporate bulk purchase rates available; please see
www.penguin.ca/corporatesales or call 1-800-810-3104, ext. 477 or 474

Acknowledgments

The authors would like to thank all of the committed professionals at Academy of the Sierras and Wellspring Camps, including Juan Alvarado Jr., Blanca Arnold, Kim Atwater, Dan Barney, Jen Barney, Nikki Beringer, Will Bettmann, Robert Burns, Ian Carter, Mark Casaus, Reynalda Ceja, Adam Chavez, Chris Clendenin, Caitlin Coffey, Elizabeth Cohen, Nicole Copillo, Nan Curry, Jessie Dean, Dawn De La Cruz, Liz Diaz, Marissa Donahue, Nick Driscoll, Todd Duncan, Garrett Earhart, Roy Felipe, Pam Fino, Brandon Fox, Dr. David Fox, John Franco, Isaac Galvan, Anna Garza, Esteban Garza, Cheryl Goh, Corrina Gonzales, John Gordon, Patricia Grogan, Chad Hickey, Beth Hockman, Katherine Howard, Amy Jackson, Shauna Johnson, Ondrej Jurik, Shannon Karian, Lev Kaye, Desiree LeGrande, Jennifer Lucas, Ryan Madamba, JoAnn Martinez, Elliot Morales, Kate Morley, Jane Morrison, Kate Nakonechny, John Navarro, Yadira Navarro, Frank Nieblas, Loren Pettigrew, Becky Pfeiffer, Amber Preheim, Luis Reyes, Silvia Reyes, Bob Rice, Natalie Richard, Lily Rocha, Matt Rosky, Zenaida Salinas, Patrice Sexton, Cara Simon, Kim Somma, Salem Starks, Mary Steward, Fida Taha, Anthony "Buff" Taylor, Cheryl Testa, Lora Tilson, Fernando Trevino, Blake Van Der Schaaf, Art Vargas, Art Vargas Jr., Ruben Vela, Michael Veredas, Annise

Weaver, Deb Sweeney Whitmore, Jeremy Whitworth, Lynn Wilson, Josh Winnecour, John Wright, Rachel Yudin, Steve Zook, and Natalie Zuniga.

AOS has many strong connections to the local San Joaquin Valley community. Steven Debuskey and Dr. Side Xi of Tulare County Health and Human Services Agency provide invaluable support to our students.

We'd also like to thank a number of people at Aspen Education Group and CRC Health Group for all their assistance over the years in creating and supporting Healthy Living Academies, especially Vera Appleyard, Elliot Sainer, Jim Dredge, Teresa Potter, Mark Hobbins, Barry Karlin, Ruth Moore, Howard Brown, Kristin Hayes, Dana Stein, JoAnn Malone, Dennis Antonetti, Tani Weiner, Jodi Falco, David Terbest, Lori Shannon, Jennifer Sedivy, Isabel Rivera, Nena Gantan, Norma Alvarado, Donna Montague, Brian Becher, Jasmine Barajas, Mary Ann Garcia, Randy Christopher, Shannon Sejkora, Rich Lam, Moriah Capan, Ingrid Martinez, Josephine Balzano, Scott Benes, John Vinaccia, and Thomas Hopkins, along with Sue Crowell, Bo Turner, and Mark Dorenfeld. Special thanks to Gil Hallows, for welcoming Ryan Craig to Aspen and helping to set the stage for the creation of Healthy Living Academies.

Thanks to Dr. Vondell Clark, director of the Weight Management Program at Catawba Valley Medical Center, North Carolina, for his tale about hunter-gatherers. We also thank Dr. Peter Neiman, director of the Pediatric Obesity Clinic in Calgary, Canada, as well as Dr. Eileen Rosendahl (New York) and Dr. Rob Smith (Boston) for their passionate support of our work. We also appreciate Eileen Crowley and her dedicated colleagues from Pfizer Health Solutions for collaborating with us in many ways.

Louis Yuhasz deserves special thanks and admiration for his tireless work on behalf of Louie's Kids, a private foundation helping many overweight children and their families change their lives.

Tina Laguna, the wonderful office manager at AOS, played an important role in helping to coordinate various aspects of this project.

Dara Obbard, wife of AOS executive director Phil Obbard, moved from New York City to Reedley, California, in order to help make AOS possible.

Many thanks to Paul Bresnick of Paul Bresnick Literary Agency for taking what was only a concept and helping us form it into this book.

The Scientific Advisory Board of Healthy Living Academies has been invaluable in helping ensure that every aspect of the program at Academy of the Sierras is scientifically based. Members of the advisory board are:

Dr. Jarol Boan, Georgia Kostas, Dr. Wolfgang Siegfried, Dr. Melinda Sothern, Dr. Dennis Styne, and Dr. Denise Wilfley.

Special thanks to chef Erin Gaughan for her innovative recipes and meal plan. Also making key contributions to these sections were Sharon Boyd, food service director at AOS, David Burns, director of operations, and Sarah Olliges, food service director and culinary instructor at AOS North Carolina.

Dan Kirschenbaum wishes to thank his colleagues at the Center for Behavioral Medicine and Sport Psychology in Chicago, particularly Sue Shrifter-Fialkow, Sherry Hirsch, and Dr. John Anderson, for their encouragement of his work at Health Living Academies; he also greatly appreciates his family's patience and support about this project, including his wonderful wife, Sue Payne, and his always loving children, Alex, Max, and Rosie.

Finally, special thanks to our researchers, without whom we would not have managed to incorporate the stories of our alumni. Jackie Windfelt, former nutrition instructor at AOS, Wellspring Adventure Camp, and Wellspring Adventure Camp California; Eileen McKeever, former activities coordinator at AOS; Chris D'Andrea, former behavioral coach at Wellspring Adventure Camp California, and now a behavioral coach at AOS; and Laurel Waterman, who may not have known the students as they transformed their lives, but who feels as if she knows them now.

We dedicate this book to the students at Academy of the Sierras and campers at Wellspring Camps who have changed their lives in so many remarkable ways; to the dedicated, committed professionals at AOS and Wellspring; and, finally, to the parents of all of our students and campers. They've done something truly remarkable: realized the importance of helping their overweight children make radical changes in their lives and trusted us to help them in that journey. We honor this trust and aspire to earn it every single day.

We also dedicate this book to Ryan Craig's wife, Yahlin Chang; she was not only our editor and guide but made many sacrifices in the early years of AOS, including but not limited to sleeping on the floor of an electrical closet while six months pregnant. Time after time, Yahlin has demonstrated the persistence and dedication that our alumni hope to achieve.

Contents

Foreword

In September 2005, Ryan Craig, one of the founders of the Academy of the Sierras, asked me if I'd be interested in coming out to California to get involved with the school. I had known Ryan for years, ever since we met in the first week of my freshman year at Yale. I distinctly recall being impressed by his diligence, initiative, and doggedness, always coupled with sensitivity and good humor. After college we stayed in touch and I was aware that Ryan was developing an interest in education and the issue of childhood obesity.

I first learned about AOS early in 2004. At the time I was working in the New York office of a major manufacturer of weight-loss products. Ryan called to get my thoughts on his idea: a boarding school for weight loss. I gave him my feedback, as well as that of the dietitians with whom I worked. And by August 2004, when my wife and I visited Ryan at his home in Los Angeles, he was busy commuting to and from the Reedley, California, campus of what was about to become, one month later, the world's first boarding school for overweight teens.

Over the next year, Ryan kept his friends apprised of the growing successes of AOS and its sister program, Wellspring Camps. In early August 2005, he let us know that AOS would be the focus of an upcoming episode of *Dateline NBC*. My wife and I watched and were both impressed and moved—my wife was moved to tears. The approach simply made much more sense than limiting one's carbohydrates or drinking a diet shake for lunch each day. And through *Dateline* I was finally able to appreciate how AOS was changing the lives of so many young people. When Ryan reached out to me one month later, I was ready to jump.

Ryan sent me information on a weight-loss program that had been developed by Dan Kirschenbaum. Dr. Kirschenbaum, a psychologist and professor at Northwestern University Medical School, had spent the preceding thirty years conducting extensive research in the fields of sport psychology and weight loss, and was widely published and highly respected by his peers. Unlike diet programs I had been exposed to in my then-current position, his work pushed a simple and direct approach to weight loss, with three primary behavioral goals:

1. Consume a very low-fat diet—20 grams of fat or fewer each day.
2. Be physically active each and every day. Aim for at least ten thousand steps a day, tracked with a pedometer.
3. Self-monitor the food you eat and your steps with the help of a journal, each and every day.

That's it. No deprivation, no convoluted rules, no bacon instead of bread; this was an approach that emphasized a "healthy obsession" to turn participants into long-term weight controllers. What's more, this approach had already been used successfully by thousands of people to lose and control their weight—including all of the students at AOS.

When I set foot on the campus of AOS for the first time, I was overwhelmed by the scope of my potential mission there: meeting the needs of over one hundred students and staff, controlling the adolescent energy that was shooting off in every direction (for better or worse), and coping with the other challenges of running a one-of-a-kind program still in its infancy. Within a few days, however, my initial concerns were swept aside by my fascination with the students: their stories, their struggles, and the positive changes so many of them were undergoing as they began to transform physically. It was then that I met some of the students you'll read about in this book for the first time—Terry H., Jill R., and Lauren E.—each tackling their emotional and weight issues head-on. Taken with them and with the dedication of the AOS staff, I began to realize that I not only wanted to be involved but that through AOS I really *could* make a positive contribution to the lives of these students.

At AOS, we ask a lot of our students. AOS is not a spa. It is not a fat camp. We don't run students ragged and we don't dictate their food choices. We teach them hard skills to help them through the stages of weight control—skills that can be applied and reapplied throughout their lives in many settings and in many ways. With a population of one hundred students, on any given day you can find students at all different stages, from honeymoon and frustration to acceptance. For every student who has slipped into the frustration stage, there is another student in honeymoon, and yet another who has reached acceptance. Often, students cycle through these stages more than once. Our focus is on helping students build the skills and coping mechanisms they will need to control their weight for the rest of their lives, not just while they are enrolled at AOS. As our outcome data demonstrates, and as you'll read in the words of AOS students themselves, we've had tremendous success.

You may have seen or read about AOS before—perhaps on our website, on CNN or *Dr. Phil,* or maybe in *People, USA Today*, or the *Washington Post*. Many local and national media outlets have done a good job of telling part of the story of the school. But we are excited about this opportunity to share not only more of the personal stories of our students but also the specifics of the plan that has yielded such impressive results.

AOS opened up its second campus in North Carolina in February 2007. Together with our summer programs, Wellspring Camps, we have had the opportunity to work with over a thousand young people and their families. Families play a crucial role in the long-term success of our students. Each is a smaller community of support that mirrors the larger community at AOS. Often, by the time they find AOS, parents have burned out on every other weight-loss approach for their child they found—sometimes including surgery—to no avail. As the mother of Terry H., one of the students profiled in this book, said, "I can say for sure that AOS gave my son a second chance on life. It saved his life."

The book you're holding tells the stories of dozens of AOS families like this and shares how they did it—how each of these amazing long-term weight controllers lost forty, sixty, even one hundred pounds on the program and, more important, kept it off for almost two years and counting. With their help, you'll now learn how your family can use the Sierras Solution to achieve the same noble and empowering goal.

Mens et Salvere,

Phil Obbard
Executive Director
Academy of the Sierras

PART 1

The Sierras Solution Philosophy

Chapter 1

The Sierras Solution: A Scientifically Based Approach to Help Kids Lose Weight

You probably wish it were you.

You wish you could take the place of your teen, your son or daughter with twenty, forty, or even more extra pounds to lose. You wish you were the one who had to face the taunts, the ridicule, the humiliation of clothes that don't fit, the extra perspiration and awkwardness in gym class. You feel their pain, and you wish you could help them.

If your son or daughter struggles with obesity, you may fear that your child will never lose the weight. In desperation, you may have already tried to encourage your child to slim down. You may have taken her to Weight Watchers meetings, bought diet books, or stocked up on bars, shakes, or other "meal replacements." You might have tried acupuncture or even questionable weight-loss supplements. Perhaps you've pleaded, pretended to ignore the problem, tried scolding or even paying your child to eat less and exercise more. Yet, after all of your efforts, your child is still over-weight, starting to falter socially, and, most tragically, may have stopped turning to you for support because she believes you've become just another person who judges her for her weight.

You may feel powerless to help your child change, but there is hope. You can do something. You can create an environment that will support your child's health as well as your own. You can work with your child to replace bad habits with good ones. You *can* help your child lose the weight and change his or her life, forever.

We know, because we've done it ourselves. As the founders of the Academy of the Sierras, the first year-round boarding school for overweight and obese kids, we've seen students lose a dramatic amount of weight and fundamentally change their lifestyles. We call our program the Sierras Solution, and it can work for your family, too.

The Obesity Epidemic Hits Home

The news media is full of shocking reports about the childhood obesity epidemic. Maybe you think that "epidemic" is too strong a word. But being overweight is undeniably a health problem, and when the incidence of any health problem skyrockets in a relatively short period of time, an epidemic is at hand.

Right now, more than one out of every three kids is overweight, or about 27 million kids in the United States and Canada. And one out of every six kids is obese—more than four times the rate of forty years ago.

Change in Childhood Overweight and Obesity

Year	% of Children with BMI 85%+	% of Children with BMI 95%+
1963–1970	16.7%	4.0%
1971–1974	21.6%	7.0%
1976–1980	24.5%	11.0%
1988–1994	29.0%	11.0%
1999–2002	31.0%	16.0%
2007	Estimated at 34%	Estimated at 17%

Yet, despite these large and growing numbers, many doctors don't provide their overweight young patients with useful treatment options. (Some doctors prefer not to raise the issue at all.) This systemic denial is largely due to the speed with which the epidemic has evolved. When most physicians practicing today were trained, pediatric obesity was not on the radar screen of medical schools or teaching hospitals. Quite simply, they just don't know what to do.

But we must do something. Overweight or obesity in a child or an adult is a health issue that can be treated. It should not be regarded as something your daughter may grow out of. She may, but it's unlikely. In fact, it's less likely to resolve itself than many other health issues that we routinely diagnose and aggressively treat. Being overweight as a child, adolescent, or young adult raises the risk of developing a number of debilitating and life-threatening physical and emotional conditions.

EXCESS WEIGHT IS PHYSICALLY DEVASTATING

Overweight children and teens are at significantly greater risk of developing immediate health problems such as hypertension, insulin resistance and diabetes, orthopedic issues, and (in girls) polycystic ovarian syndrome. They are also very likely to become *more* overweight—not less—as adults.

- A study conducted by Dr. Philip Nader and colleagues at the University of California, San Diego, School of Medicine found that children who are overweight at any point before age five are more than five times more likely than other children to be overweight at age twelve.
- Other studies have shown that overweight adolescents are twenty times more likely than other adolescents to become obese young adults. Approximately 75 percent of obese children become obese adults.

Obesity in adulthood can often mean the difference between life and death. As the obesity epidemic has spiraled out of control, researchers have correlated obesity with practically every major disease category, including:

- Diabetes
- Coronary heart disease
- Hypertension
- Stroke
- Osteoarthritis
- Gallstones

- Various cancers, including breast cancer, cervical cancer, uterine cancer, colon cancer, esophageal cancer, pancreatic cancer, kidney cancer, and prostate cancer
- Pulmonary conditions (think sleep apnea)
- Liver diseases
- Gynecological abnormalities
- Skin conditions
- Gout
- Cataracts
- Pancreatitis

True, we rarely see kids with conditions such as cataracts or cancer. These diseases take time to develop, and often will, as a result of obesity.

While many overweight and obese kids aren't burdened with these potentially fatal physical problems—yet—most take a beating in another sense: psychologically.

EXCESS WEIGHT IS EMOTIONALLY DEVASTATING

According to many studies, kids consistently view their overweight peers as "lazy, lying, cheating, sloppy, dirty, ugly, and stupid." Other studies have correlated obesity in adolescence and young adulthood to failure to complete high school, failure to attend college, failure to graduate from college, failure to enter into a relationship and get married, and an increased likelihood of occupying a lower socioeconomic level as an adult.

Obese children are almost always socially stigmatized and very often suffer from serious emotional and psychological disorders, such as depression, anxiety disorders, and adjustment disorders. In a startling study, researchers from the University of California, San Diego, in 2003 found that obese children rate their quality of life as low as young cancer patients do. In this study, 106 obese children ages 5 to 18 who had been referred to a hospital were asked to rate their physical, academic, emotional, and social well-being. Compared to a control group of children in a normal weight range, the obese children were five times more likely to report a low quality of life. In particular, the emotional, social, and psychological states of the obese children mapped most closely with those of young cancer patients. Both categories of children had trouble keeping up with peers at school and participating in activities, and both groups were teased and ostracized by classmates. Even the researchers were surprised by the results.

You want to protect your children. The last thing you'd ever want is for them to experience this kind of pain. But how can you help them when all factors seem to conspire against their success? That's exactly the problem we set out to solve when we created Academy of the Sierras (AOS).

We Started with Science

Some health-care policymakers think overweight in young people is a lost cause. They believe society's primary focus should be on preventing kids who aren't overweight from becoming overweight, given that it's so difficult for overweight kids to lose weight, and even more difficult to control it over a long period of time.

As educators and researchers, we experienced the childhood obesity epidemic firsthand. We saw the toll it was taking on our children and that it wasn't going away. Dan Kirschenbaum was a professor at Northwestern University Medical School in Chicago who had been researching and treating obese adults and children for three decades. Ryan Craig was based in New York City and was a leader in the field of education, serving on the boards of many organizations and companies serving children. And Lisa Tjelmeland was a social worker in St. Louis working with children with a range of emotional and behavioral issues. We knew that the problem was so pervasive, with so many moving pieces, that we needed a fresh approach. Rather than give up on an entire generation of kids, we were very confident we could produce an effective solution.

Led by Dan Kirschenbaum, AOS was founded by a group of scientists with the backing of Aspen Education Group, a leading organization of therapeutic schools and residential programs focused on behavioral change in children, adolescents, and young adults. Aspen operates thirty-six programs in fifteen states and the United Kingdom and serves more than four thousand children every year. These boarding schools and programs vary widely in nature, but what they have in common is a deep commitment to working closely with adolescents in emotionally safe, therapeutic environments to change behavior successfully. We'd seen how a dedicated program could turn lives around for kids with other emotional and behavioral issues, including substance abuse and acting out. We knew the model would help overweight kids as well.

When we opened our first campus in California in September 2004, our first class of seven students attended grades eight through twelve; now we have one hundred students at this campus. Our second campus opened in February 2007 in North Carolina, with a first class of eleven students. Now, we enroll up to fifty students in grades six through ten.

Students typically enroll for about two semesters, or nine months. The longest any student has been enrolled is sixteen months. A child wouldn't go through the entire four years of high school at Academy of the Sierras. There's no need for that, because most of our students return to a normal weight range in nine months.

We've seen dramatic results—students have lost twenty, forty, eighty, even a hundred and twenty or more pounds while at our school. But what's been most gratifying to us is seeing how sustainable the program is. After the kids leave AOS, they continue to lose weight and, most important, maintain their weight loss and their long-term commitment to a much healthier lifestyle.

When we saw those results—that teenagers could maintain their weight loss out in the real world, far from the confines of the school—we knew that the core principles of the program could help everyone. We knew that other families could learn and adopt the core principles and see those kinds of changes in their own homes. And once we realized that, we were determined to share the program more broadly, so that those who might never have the opportunity to come to AOS could still benefit from the program that had changed so many lives.

How the Sierras Solution Is Different

The Academy of the Sierras was founded by a group of leading weight-control scientists. When we started, we made a commitment to develop a program that employs every tool known to science to be effective for weight loss and long-term weight control. We've based our approach exclusively on credible, peer-reviewed studies, the work of thousands of researchers at universities and hospitals around the world. As a result, AOS is the only weight-loss program for children that takes full advantage of the decades of scientifically established research on weight control.

Our primary goal is to help children become what we call "long-term weight controllers" (LTWCs). We do it through a combination of diet management, activity, education, training, and cognitive-behavioral therapy. At the core of our approach is the recognition that obesity is a highly complex problem with three main facets.

First of all, *obesity is clearly biological*. Two children raised in the same house by the same parents and exhibiting largely the same behaviors can diverge wildly in terms of their weight. At AOS, we frequently hear from parents about the older or younger sibling who is "as thin as a rail." We help kids both recognize and accept this reality, so they can move on to crafting a program that takes their "unjust" situation into account rather than denying it exists. We'll talk more about the biological factor in chapter 2.

Second of all, *obesity is clearly environmental*, as evidenced by the chart on page 4. In one generation, the environment for diet and activity has changed radically. This is the only explanation for the epidemic. Our biology hasn't changed in thirty years—it doesn't change in thirty thousand years, let alone thirty. While we can't reverse these changes in the outside world, we do help kids recognize the traps and craft a personal environment that's more supportive to their long-term weight-control efforts. We'll discuss this more in chapter 2 as well.

Finally, *obesity is clearly behavioral*. Many lifestyle habits that lead to weight gain are unconscious, yet can be devastating to personal health. A thirteen-year-old girl with an extremely compromised biology, living in today's fast-food society, *can* successfully control her weight if she adopts a set of specific behaviors. If she doesn't, she will become overweight or obese. We can change only a few aspects of our biology, and we have limited influence over our environment. But we have tremendous control over our behavior. This is the cornerstone tenet of the Sierras Solution plan.

From our experience with other educational programs, we've seen that while anyone can change, children are particularly adaptable and adept at changing their life course. The Sierras Solution will help you help your child (and you) master the three scientifically proven lifestyle behaviors—which we call the three Simple Changes—that will lead to a new path toward significant weight loss and lifelong weight control. The three simple, yet effective, directives in the Sierras Solution are:

Defining "Overweight" in Kids

Not long ago, AOS received an e-mail from a parent that said:

> My child has a BMI at the 92nd percentile for her height and age. While this is technically labeled as "at risk for being overweight," I am very concerned about her happiness and self-image. I am exploring many options currently and would like more information about your program. Thank you.

Researchers define overweight and obesity with the body mass index, a measure of your weight in kilograms divided by the square of your height in meters. But why would a child with a body mass index at the 92nd percentile for her height and age be called "at risk for being overweight" instead of just "overweight"?

BMI is measured differently in children and adults. Both age and gender must be taken into account for children, because boys and girls are still growing and have different percentages of body fat. An eleven-year-old girl who is 4 feet 11 inches and 140 pounds should be viewed differently from a fifty-year-old woman of the same height and weight. But while the BMI benchmark for adults is very clear (BMI over 25 is overweight; BMI over 30 is obese), the benchmarks for growing children are BMI percentage: being above the 95th percentile BMI for age and gender is defined as "overweight," and a BMI score in the 85th to 95th percentile is defined as "at risk of overweight."

According to this definition, there is no such thing as an obese child. But isn't it appropriate to apply the term "obese" to the heaviest kids, in the same way we do for adults? What about the three-hundred-pound seventeen-year-old boy whose doctor says he is "overweight." When he turns eighteen, does he become "obese" without gaining one more pound?

Health-care professionals outside the United States use the terms "obese" and "overweight" for young people just as they do for adults. American doctors have not been comfortable with the idea of telling kids they are obese. They fear the term is judgmental and harsh and will possibly lead to confrontations with upset parents. The 2002 National Health and Nutrition Examination Survey revealed that only 36.7 percent of overweight kids had been told by a doctor or other health-care professional that they were overweight.

(continued)

Kids hear much worse than "obese" in the schoolyard. Hearing from a doctor that they are obese could play an important role in establishing a foundation for change. If we're going to solve a problem, let's start by being honest about it. In this book, just as at AOS, we use the terms "overweight" and "obese."

- Eat as little fat as possible, with a goal of fewer than 20 grams of fat a day.
- Be as active as possible and wear a pedometer. Aim for at least ten thousand steps per day.
- Self-monitor—keep a record of your eating and exercise—every day or at least 75 percent of the time.

We'll talk more about the science behind these guidelines, and how you can implement them in your family life, in part 2 of the book. For now, let's take a look at how these three Simple Changes have made all the difference to our students, and they can change your child's life, too.

Our Results Speak for Themselves

Our commitment to science didn't end with the creation of the AOS program. On the contrary, that commitment extended to evaluating our own students' outcomes. We wanted to be sure our program produced real, clinically significant results.

Just as other researchers do, we organized, staged, and analyzed our students' experiences in order to provide clinically and statistically significant results about their experience on the AOS program. With three years behind us, we now know that our program's outcomes are unprecedented in the history of research on childhood overweight and obesity. We are proud to say that research shows no other program has worked as effectively as the Sierras Solution.

The first study was completed in the late spring of 2006 for the first class of students to graduate from AOS. These fifteen students, who completed the program in June 2005, were about fifteen years old (on average) and averaged 100 percent overweight when they entered AOS, meaning that they were twice as heavy as they should have been. The average student was enrolled for thirty-one weeks (about seven months).

The average student lost eighty-one pounds over the seven months. At the beginning, all of them lost weight faster; the weight loss slowed down as they had less and less weight to lose. But the average for the seven months was close to three pounds per week, which is about three times better than the average of other weight-loss programs reported in articles published in peer-reviewed scientific journals.

We were delighted, but not very surprised. After all, AOS is the first weight-loss program to keep "patients" in a controlled environment for such a long period of time. Some experts expected us to achieve this record level of weight loss. The big question was what would happen when these students returned home. Sixty percent of these students had returned to a normal weight range at AOS. Many of them didn't have much weight left to lose when they went home. We watched them closely to see what would happen next.

In the spring of 2006, ten months after students had left the Academy, we found something truly remarkable. Some regained some weight, but an equal number continued to lose more weight. On average, AOS alumni retained 100 percent of the weight loss achieved at AOS.

Of course, we are overjoyed with these results. And we're even more gratified because we've seen the program work in alternative settings as well. We also run four- to eight-week summer programs, called Wellspring Camps, and our results there are equally remarkable. While some campers may lose as many as fifty pounds because of the shorter time frame, few campers are able to return to a normal weight range at camp. After losing fifteen to thirty pounds at camp, most campers are still overweight—some very overweight. But campers who attended Wellspring had not only maintained their weight loss six to nine months later—on average they had gone on to lose an additional five to eight pounds. These results further confirmed our conviction that the program can work in the real world as well, for everyone in the family. The Sierras Solution's simple and sustainable guidelines can be followed by all family members interested in living a healthy lifestyle—regardless of whether they have a weight problem.

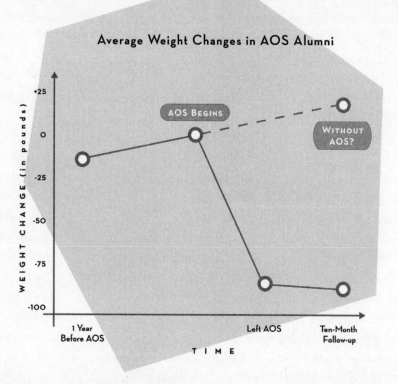

Average Weight Changes in AOS Alumni

WEIGHT CHANGE (in pounds)

+25

0

-25

-50

-75

-100

AOS Begins

WITHOUT AOS?

1 Year
Before AOS

Left AOS

Ten-Month
Follow-up

TIME

How to Use this Book

If you're reading this book, you're obviously invested in helping your child tackle his or her weight issue. We know that this is a tough process, fraught with all kinds of emotional and physical challenges, perhaps for you as well as your child. We ask that you approach this program with total honesty—which is the foundation of the AOS program—and see it as a huge opportunity for growth and intimacy for your entire family. Your child needs your faith, understanding, and support. You are asking him or her to place trust in you as a partner in this noble goal. Do your best to be worthy of that trust by facing your own issues and acknowledging the roles you all play in losing the weight.

At the school, we have the benefit of creating an environment that surrounds and supports the student's weight-loss efforts from day one. You can re-create that tremendous advantage in your own home in several ways. First, read part 1, to get a firm handle on the background of the Sierras Solution program. In chapter 2, you'll learn more about how your child gained the weight and what makes it so difficult to lose. Read chapter 3 to learn how you can set your child on the right path and how your involvement is so crucial to his or her success.

Then discuss the program with your teen. Talk about what you've learned. See if he or she is willing to join with you and make the commitment to lose weight.

Once you have a commitment, set a start date for your program. Read part 2 together, to get a clear picture of the entire plan. Some people will find it easier to jump in and adopt the entire program all at once; others will prefer to ease into it by taking on one Simple Change a week until they've incorporated all three into their lives. One easy way to start off on the right foot is to use the complete menu plan and recipes to guide your family's eating while you're learning about the program.

As you learn about the Sierras Solution together, make it a fun partnership or, ideally, a group effort with the whole family. Do the shopping together. Clean out the pantry together. Cook the meals together. Get your child as involved in buying and preparing her food as possible. Try to make the entire journey positive, energizing, and rewarding.

Throughout the book, we'll introduce you and your child to several AOS alumni. These young people have volunteered to share writings from their journals or thoughts from earlier conversations. They reveal some of their deepest feelings of shame and frustration from when they first started the Sierras Solution program, as well as their tremendous joy in their remarkable achievements upon their transition back home and up to two years later. We believe that reading through the thoughts of the alumni is one of the best ways you and your child can understand both the practice and the promise of the Sierras Solution.

We hope you join us and give your child the chance to change his or her life the way so many AOS students have. First, we'll look at the issue of excess weight itself—where it comes from and why it is so very hard to lose. Knowing the enemy is the first step to defeating it!

Chapter 2

Why Kids Gain Weight: Understanding the Powerful Biological and Environmental Factors

The first step toward helping your child return to a normal weight for life is to develop an understanding of the challenges he or she is facing. Let's start with this question: What makes losing weight and keeping it off so difficult?

Is it biology—your genes, fat cells, hormones, enzymes and metabolic rate, the amount of energy your body requires to simply stay alive at rest?

Or is it everything else—your environment, culture, family influences, habits, lifestyles, personality, and emotional functioning?

If you had to pick one primary factor that causes weight problems in kids more than any other, what would you say—is it biology, or everything else?

Parents often answer this question by invoking challenges like fast food, instant messaging, supersized portions, and busy lifestyles. If you answered the way 95 percent of AOS parents did, you would say that both answers were correct, but that "everything else" clearly has the edge over biology. That's the logical answer to the question—after all, the environment, culture, and our habits and lifestyle seem to be responsible for weight gain.

But that perfectly logical and reasonable answer isn't the best one. The greatest factor in the struggle to lose weight is *biology*.

Biology Can Be Unfair

If you have one overweight child and another who has never struggled with his or her weight, as most AOS families do, you may already understand that biology can dramatically affect weight status. Consider the experience of fifteen-year-old Dan K. (whose profile is featured on page 54). Dan and his fraternal twin brother, Sam, are very close. They hang out together, share mutual friends, and love to do things together. Their mother struggles with a substantial weight problem, but works very hard to give all of her children good lives, full of positive support and opportunities.

In contrast to Dan, Sam has never had a weight problem. He eats whatever he wants without gaining any weight. Their father loves to eat nuts, and he leaves them all over the house. When tempting foods come into the house, their mother is conscious of this physical difference between the two boys, and she sometimes tells Dan that certain treats, like Halloween candy, are "not for you."

Dan is a great sport about it; he says he "doesn't want to inconvenience" his family by complaining about these temptations. But he confesses that it's harder than he thought it would be to avoid them when they're lying around the house. Those temptations don't add a pound to his brother, but they represent a tremendous challenge to Dan's less robust metabolism.

Sam and Dan have almost identical environments, yet one became more than one hundred pounds overweight while the other remained slim. Why? Biology.

Even in two siblings from the same family, apparently minor differences between individuals can belie a tremendous variation in their ability to burn off calories. Sam and Dan share many of the same genes, but they are not identical—in some ways, they are as dissimilar metabolically as if they were from different families.

Research by Canadian psychologist Dr. Claude Bouchard at Laval University helped make this point. Dr. Bouchard and his colleagues studied twelve sets of young identical twin boys who lived in a controlled environment for one hundred days. After a baseline period of twelve days, the twins were given one thousand calories above their usual levels of intake for the next eighty-four days. Some participants gained about nine pounds but others gained almost thirty—all under virtually identical conditions. The best predictor of how much weight any one boy gained was how much his twin gained. Some twins apparently had the biological tendency to gain weight easily, whereas others did not.

If you fully understand the power of biology as a cause of this problem, you'll appreciate why becoming a successful weight controller demands considerable effort and support. Dan has to learn what is and what isn't for him in his own household. On the other hand, teens who don't have this biological handicap, like Dan's brother, Sam, don't ever have to think about it.

Developing an understanding of these biological challenges is key to helping your child start down the path of long-term weight control. Let's begin by considering the biological demands faced by our collective ancestors.

Our Hunter-Gatherer Bodies

Experts tell us that somewhere between seven thousand to ten thousand years ago humans began farming, raising crops, and keeping animals. Try to imagine what life was like in the years before that happened. Before then, humans had to hunt, fish, and forage for food. We had to stay active to stay alive. And food was not plentiful. When your tribe finally caught a deer, you gobbled it down quickly, because you were starving and because if you didn't eat it, someone else would. In your travels to find food and shelter and stay alive, you probably covered about fifty thousand steps a day.

Fast-forward to today. The average North American gets about four thousand steps per day. After a sedentary day at school (most days rarely incorporate any physical education), your child comes home to slump on the couch in front of TV, video games, or the computer—or all three. The average child spends about 4.5 hours per day in front of a screen. By the time your child turns in, he's only been active or even moving for about 1.5 hours per day—a fraction of his peer in hunter-gather times. The problem is, our bodies still "think" we are all hunter-gatherers, storing fat efficiently and resisting weight loss aggressively to safeguard against famines of short and long duration. The same biological forces that caused our ancestors to gulp down the deer meat also give us the impulse to devour extra servings of pizza in the cafeteria, or scavenge through the cupboards after getting home from school. Even more important, we were designed to move—to move a lot—for most of the day. In the few remaining countries and cultures where people still move around a great deal throughout the day, weight problems remain relatively rare. By contrast, modern American culture encourages very sedentary living. A third of American children and teens are now overweight or obese, in large part because they don't move around enough.

It's a wonder everyone isn't overweight. Yet, you undoubtedly know kids like Dan's brother, Sam. They have a diet and activity level similar to those of your overweight son or daughter and yet somehow remain slim. Despite our sedentary culture and abundance of foods, some people inherit the tendency to stay slim and some people inherit the tendency to gain weight easily. These biological factors have a pronounced impact on weight.

Biological Barriers to Weight Loss

Perhaps your children suffer the same fate—they don't eat much, and sometimes clearly less than their peers, yet they gain weight easily. We'll consider some of the details of these biological barriers in order to help you appreciate and accept their power.

When you do read about them, you might feel justifiably angry on your child's behalf. We can't tell you the number of times we've heard (and thought to ourselves), "It's just not fair." But we want you to remember one critical caveat as you read about them: *Biology is not destiny*.

Vicki M., a fourteen-year-old AOS alum who lost fifty-four pounds on the program, came to this empowering realization, and it helped her take control.

I just remember one September night a few months after leaving AOS; it was after homecoming or something. And I was, like, "If I don't control myself now, I'm gonna be put back in the same place I was before." And things have to change in my life. And I can't sit here and whine that this is my biology and this is what is meant to be for my life. I have to be happy that I have the chance to do this. So I was, like, "Get over yourself. Just do it."

If biology were fully and completely in charge, no one would ever lose weight and keep it off. Vicki refused to accept her biological limitations. Your son and daughter can do the same.

There are actually many distinct biological factors that make weight control quite difficult. Whenever people develop excess weight, at any point in their lives, their bodies become especially efficient and effective at maintaining higher-than-normal levels of fat. These biological forces include ones that begin before birth and others that develop over the years. Of the many factors, AOS students and their parents tell us that the following five biological factors have the greatest impact on their efforts and help remind them of the power of this biological foe.

> *Oh, you know you're always judged. "Oh, his mother must be driving him crazy to eat like that." But it turns out that it is genetics.*
>
> —MOTHER OF JESSE G., FIFTEEN,
>   TORONTO, CANADA
>   JESSE'S INITIAL WEIGHT LOSS:
>   EIGHTY-EIGHT POUNDS IN SIX MONTHS
>   JESSE'S SUSTAINED WEIGHT LOSS:
>   NINETY-TWO POUNDS FOR FIVE MONTHS

THE PERMANENCE OF GENES

Research shows that our genetic inheritance has a huge influence on our metabolic power and tendency to develop excess fat. In breeding studies with mice, fatter mice have been mated with other fatter mice and leaner mice with other leaner mice. Over fifteen to twenty-five generations, this can produce mice pups from the fatter matings with twice as much fat as the pups from the leaner matings. Research on humans shows that children born to obese parents are four times more likely to become obese than children born to lean parents.

In the twin study we mentioned earlier, in which the twelve pairs of twins were overfed for one hundred days, we saw that if one member of a twin pair gained a lot of weight, the other member of the pair did also. Other studies with twins growing up in separate households have shown similar trends: they resemble each other in weight status much more than the siblings with whom they grew up.

Why Kids Gain Weight:
Understanding the
Powerful Biological and
Environmental Factors

———

Some of us are simply born with bodies primed to gain weight easily from day one while others may resist weight gain. And just as genetics dramatically affects weight gain, it similarly affects weight regain after losing it—that's why we emphasize that kids who follow the Sierras Solution are "long-term weight controllers." Those genes, for better or worse, are with your child for life.

THE HUNGER OF FAT CELLS

We call fat cells "hungry baby sparrows" because they are so efficient at storing excess food as fat. And overweight people have many more fat cells than people who have never been overweight, up to *four times* as many of these hungry creatures (in some cases, one hundred sixty billion versus forty billion). Unfortunately, liposuction can barely make a dent, removing only a few million cells or so, because fat is intertwined in our muscles and organs.

Adding fat cells doesn't take long; some studies have shown that animals that are fed large amounts of high-fat food can permanently gain excess fat cells within one week. You can develop more at any point in your life and, once they develop, they never, ever disappear.

Why is this so important? Studies have traced where the body sends fat after eating. Apparently, for overweight and formerly overweight people, the body delivers fat into the fat cells more efficiently, perhaps directed by some of the biological devices described below. People who have never had weight problems seem to have more fat transported into muscles for use as immediate fuel.

THE HORMONES THAT *FIGHT* WEIGHT LOSS

Evolution established a number of hormones and enzymes as biological barriers against weight loss. The specifics are complex, and it's not essential that you understand the mechanics of each one, but the overall picture is daunting. We'll walk through them one by one to give you a sense of what you're up against.

Insulin

Insulin, which is stored and manufactured in special cells within the pancreas, promotes the ingestion of blood sugar (glucose) by our cells. Just as gas fuels your car, glucose fuels your cells. Some overweight people have excess insulin in their bloodstreams at all times. Their bodies can become insensitive to the insulin, rendering their insulin less efficient at getting the glucose into their cells. This is why overweight people are prone to developing type 2 diabetes—a disease in which the body can't use all of the insulin that is produced, so the glucose continues to stay in the blood. Excessive glucose in the blood creates problems throughout the body, including attaching permanently to proteins in the eyes, kidneys, and small blood vessels of various organs. These protein-glucose linkages makes those proteins function abnormally, sometimes causing critical body parts—such as the eyes, kidneys, heart, and nerve cells—to fail. Type 2 diabetes has deadly consequences because of this, shortening the juvenile diabetic's life expectancy by twenty-five years on average.

> *When I used to go out to eat, people would often say, "You should try this; you should try that." Before coming to AOS, I would say, "Yeah, I'll try all kinds of things. Give it all to me!" If something was in front of me, I wanted to eat it all. It didn't matter what it was. It could never be enough.*
>
> —Terry H., fifteen,
> Exeter, New Hampshire
> Initial weight loss:
> 305 pounds in sixteen months
> Sustained weight loss:
> 280 pounds for more than one year

To make matters worse, when people lose weight, the body's fat cells become even more sensitive to insulin. Concurrently, the muscle cells decrease their sensitivity to insulin, so the muscle cells can't use as much glucose as usual. The excess energy can then get stored quite efficiently in the highly sensitive fat cells. That's the reason several studies have shown that the increased insulin sensitivity caused by weight loss may play a role when people regain weight very readily.

LPL

Lipoprotein lipase (LPL) is an enzyme (a special chemical agent) produced in many cells. LPL stays on the walls of very small blood vessels and can become activated to transport fat in the body. During weight loss, increases in LPL occur as fat cells release their LPL into the bloodstream. By doing so, the fat cells send messages to the brain: "Get more food in us, now!" This probably increases hunger when people try to lose weight.

Why Kids Gain Weight: Understanding the Powerful Biological and Environmental Factors

—

Leptin

Leptin, a hormone discovered in 1994, is secreted by fat cells to act as a messenger between the cells and the brain, directing the amount of fat that gets stored in fat cells by affecting appetite. As fat cells shrink during weight loss, these cells decrease the amount of leptin they release into the bloodstream. Lower circulating levels of leptin can increase appetite and in turn contribute to weight regain.

Ghrelin

The hormone ghrelin is one of the body's strongest known appetite stimulants. Ghrelin is produced in the stomach and is associated with the size of the stomach. One study found that when weight controllers lost 17 percent of their body weight, their levels of ghrelin rose by 24 percent. Weight-loss surgery (such as the gastric bypass) decreases the size of the stomach and therefore decreases ghrelin substantially. With less appetite (due to decreased ghrelin), those who undergo these surgeries don't have to fight the ghrelin battle. Of course, with a complication rate that is somewhere between 20 and 40 percent, and with a 1 percent mortality rate, gastric bypass surgery is not an easy choice to make.

Adiponectin

Adiponectin is a protein secreted by fat cells (like leptin) that helps insulin direct blood sugar from the bloodstream into your body's cells. Unfortunately, the more fat cells and larger fat cells a person has, the less adiponectin the fat cells secrete. Less adiponectin means that overweight people have a greater propensity to direct blood sugar into fat cells rather than using it for energy.

Between adiponectin, ghrelin, leptin, LPL, and insulin, you can see that the overweight body powerfully resists weight loss.

THE DECREASING CALORIE BURN OF ADAPTIVE THERMOGENESIS

When weight controllers attempt to lose weight and reduce the amount of food they consume, their bodies have the capability to switch into a very efficient mode. Remember the plight of the hunter-gatherers, whose bodies we have inherited. To survive, their bodies had to make adjustments when they couldn't catch a deer in a particular week. Adaptive thermogenesis allowed their bodies to survive on fewer calories and slowed down their metabolism during times when adequate amounts of food simply weren't available.

That's why simply reducing calorie intake by, say, five hundred calories a day may not promote any weight loss. The weight controller's body may use adaptive thermogenesis to switch from its normal mode to a much more efficient, calorie-saving mode. But you can reverse this effect by moving more than usual and exercising every day. Exercise makes it possible for weight controllers to lose weight by bypassing the effects of adaptive thermogenesis.

THE BODY'S DESIRE FOR A WEIGHT SET POINT

Don't forget—our hunter-gatherer body has no idea we are hip deep in plentiful food, so its main objective is to stay alive and not let us starve. As a weight controller tries to lose weight, his or her body uses adaptive thermogenesis to become efficient. The body also relies on various hormones and enzymes (like insulin, leptin, LPL) to make it difficult to lose weight and keep it off. Fat cells themselves, including their unusual ability to expand in size and number, also contribute to this problem.

The set-point concept summarizes all of these effects, making it clear that weight controllers are stuck in bodies that use a variety of biological forces to resist weight loss. Just as leptin has been a recent discovery, undoubtedly there are other biological mechanisms that contribute to the body's desire to maintain an excessive amount of fat. Research with animals has shown that very overweight rats and mice show similar tendencies to "defend" (or "set") the amount of fat in their bodies at a very high level.

Unfortunately, part of this defense (or set point) includes a tendency for the bodies of overweight people to respond more dramatically to the sight, the smell, and even the thought of tempting foods. A study by Dr. William Johnson and associates at the University of Mississippi Medical School showed that overweight participants, compared to their lean counterparts, increased their insulin responses not just by eating bacon and eggs but by seeing and smelling them—and even by *thinking* about bacon and eggs. They even drooled more than leaner participants, indicating just how great their desire was to consume more food in order to decrease the levels of these appetite-stimulating hormones in their bloodstream. This oversecretion of insulin and digestive enzymes is thought to help "defend" high weights even more effectively.

Environmental Barriers to Weight Loss

Now let's get back to "everything else," or the environment, which experts have labeled "obesogenic"—meaning that becoming obese is almost a natural consequence of living in modern North America, and increasingly other developed countries.

While biology rules, environment also matters a lot. To give you a sense of the importance of environment on weight, consider this: overweight people are more likely to have overweight pets than people who are in a normal weight range. There's definitely no genetic relationship there!

Biology is undoubtedly the primary reason losing weight is so difficult. But biology is not responsible for the epidemic of childhood overweight and obesity. Our biology hasn't changed in the past generation. What has changed is the environment.

Consider these eight environmental factors that have done a number on our kids' ability to stay lean.

SUPERSIZED PORTIONS

A traditional burger, fries, and Coke at McDonald's used to contain 627 calories and 19 grams of fat. Today, the standard combo has 1,805 calories and 84 grams of fat—nearly triple the calories and more than quadruple the fat!

A standard serving of Coca-Cola used to be 6.5 ounces—90 calories. Today, the standard serving is 20 ounces and packs 250 calories.

Snickers use to come in one size—1.1 ounces or 210 calories. Today, the Snickers "Big One"—3.7 ounces—satisfies with 500 calories.

The list goes on and on, from fast food and snacks to traditional restaurant and grocery items. Why have portions been supersized? Like all companies, food and beverage companies—packaged goods and restaurants alike—aim to maximize their profits. And over the past generation, they've found they can make more money through larger portions.

Here's how it works: If you're McDonald's and you charge $1.00 for a small order of fries, $1.40 for a medium fries, and $1.80 for a large fries, which item will you make the most money on? Except for a few extra pennies for the larger carton and additional potatoes, each serving costs you the same amount to produce. The largest expense, the overhead—the physical restaurant itself, the franchise fee, the labor, electricity—costs the same regardless of whether the customer buys a small or a large. While McDonald's may make 20 cents of profit on the small fries, it makes 50 cents on the medium and 80 cents on the large. So, if you're McDonald's, you're going to try to sell as many large fries as possible.

Unfortunately for us, we've gotten into a bad habit of believing that we're getting a "good deal" by spending a little bit more to get a lot more food. In fact, it's a good deal for the company. It's a bad deal for us.

MEALS PREPARED BY OTHER PEOPLE

With our fast-paced lives, we're also eating more and more meals away from home, prepared by someone else. In 1975, Americans ate 25 percent of their meals outside of the home. In 2007, it's estimated that Americans will probably eat out for nearly 50 percent of their meals. Restaurant meals account for about 50 cents out of every dollar Americans spend on food—and half of that is spent at fast-food eateries such as McDonald's, Burger King, Wendy's, and Pizza Hut.

Eating out is convenient. It's fun. But the trade-off is control. By going out to eat, we're giving up control of ingredients, method of preparation, and portion size. As very few restaurants put your weight and health at the top of their agenda, compromises are made along each of these dimensions—compromises you probably wouldn't make if you ate at home and retained control. The result is we're eating more high-fat, calorie-dense foods.

What Is Calorie Density?

Calorie density refers to the ratio of calories in a food to the mass and/or volume of that food. Chocolate has a very high calorie density: 160 calories per ounce. Water has zero calorie density—0 calories, no matter how large the serving size!

Calorie density is important because most people will stop eating, or at least eat less, when they're full. And the mass or volume of food in your stomach plays a key role in signaling whether you're full.

The Sierras Solution makes fantastic use of low-calorie-density foods. We love foods with high water content such as soups, stews, vegetables, and fruits. While many fruits have more calories than most vegetables, they still have a relatively low calorie density because of their high water content.

Calorie density is one of the reasons we advocate minimizing fat intake. While both carbohydrate and protein measure 4 calories per gram, 1 gram of fat has 9 calories. This means that fats are more than twice as calorie-dense as carbohydrates and proteins. When you cut out fats, you inherently lower the calorie density of your diet, which automatically helps you reduce your total caloric intake.

THE ECONOMIC AND PSYCHOLOGICAL POWER OF ADVERTISING

Food and beverage companies aren't deliberately trying to make our children fat. They're trying to generate good returns for their shareholders. But it turns out that a good way to do that has been to market large portions of high-fat, calorie-dense foods to our kids.

Food and beverage marketers spend more than $15 billion per year in the United States and Canada promoting their products to kids. A recent Kaiser Family Foundation study found that eight- to twelve-year-olds see 7,600 food ads per year, 40 percent of which are for candy, snacks, or fast food. And those ads work. Multiple studies have shown that children who are exposed to advertising ask their parents to buy high-fat, calorie-dense foods and sugary beverages. It's what kids want. It's what they pester you to buy. It's what they buy themselves.

Not surprisingly, researchers have correlated television viewing and exposure to ads with a reduction in consumption of fruits and vegetables, presumably corresponding to an increase in the consumption of less nutritious foods. Every additional hour of television per day results in one fewer serving of fruits and vegetables every six days.

Advertising for soft drinks in the United States alone has increased much faster in recent years than other advertising, going from $541 million in 1995 to $800 million in 1999—an almost 50 percent increase in four years. In the past generation, the percentage of American children who drink soda increased from 37 percent to over 60 percent, and average daily consumption among children who drink soda increased from 14 to 21 ounces.

And where are the health promotion messages? Teenagers see one public service announcement promoting fitness or nutrition for every 130 food ads. In their remarkable 2004 book, *Food Fight*, Drs. Kelly Brownell and Katherine Horgen of Yale University pointed out a basic inequity: "At its peak, the 5-A-Day fruit and vegetable program from the National Cancer Institute had $2 million for promotion. This is one-fifth of the $10 million spent annually to advertise Altoids mints."

It's simply not a level playing field.

> *PE was always difficult. You don't want to change in the locker room, really, you don't want to go out and try and participate because you're going to be the last one, and you're not as capable as everyone else.*
>
> —LAUREN S.,* FIFTEEN,
> CALABASAS, CALIFORNIA
> INITIAL WEIGHT LOSS:
> FIFTY POUNDS IN FOUR MONTHS
> SUSTAINED WEIGHT LOSS:
> SIXTY-FOUR POUNDS FOR MORE THAN
> ONE YEAR
> (*SEE LAUREN'S PROFILE ON PAGE 32.)

THE STEADY DECLINE OF PHYS ED

Another important factor is the near elimination of physical education in most school districts. Forced by federal and state governments to focus on math and reading test scores, many schools have had to cut electives, such as art, music, and physical education, to accommodate resulting time and resource constraints. Today, only 8 percent of American elementary schools, 6 percent of middle schools, and 5 percent of high schools provide daily physical education. Many of our students report that gym is rare, and even when they have it, they are often eager and able to refrain from participating.

THE DOWNSIDE OF DIGITAL ENTERTAINMENT

Admittedly, a generation ago, some kids would return home after school and watch television. Most of the time, though, kids would engage in some level of physical activity—an organized sport, playing with other kids on the block, or even just climbing trees in the backyard.

Today, average daily television viewing is up by more than 30 percent since 1980. Almost half of all children ages eight to sixteen watch three to five hours of television a day. Television is certainly a major contributor to childhood obesity, and many studies have correlated television viewing to overweight in childhood and obesity in adulthood.

But that's not the whole story, especially for today's preteens and teenagers. Their digital indulgences are the computer and related devices, like the Sony PlayStation and the Xbox. The favorite after-school activity has become logging on to MySpace while instant-messaging friends, followed by a marathon PlayStation session.

Not only do these activities result in a huge reduction in calories burned compared with the active games and sports their counterparts played twenty-seven years ago, they also lend themselves to snacking. Now we have a double-whammy: reduced caloric expenditure and increased caloric intake.

THE CAR-CENTRIC NORTH AMERICAN LIFESTYLE

In the United States and Canada, only 10 percent of city travel occurs on foot or by bicycle. In relatively newer cities, like Los Angeles, Atlanta, and Dallas, where people rely on cars for almost everything, fewer than 5 percent of trips involve biking or walking. In contrast, at least 40 percent of trips in urban areas of Austria, Denmark, the Netherlands, and Sweden are made by bicycle or on foot. People bicycle or walk for at least 30 percent of their urban trips in France, Germany, and Switzerland.

This tendency in the United States and Canada extends to how our children travel to school. Thirty years ago, most children would walk or bike to school. Ninety percent of kids who lived within a mile of school would walk or bike. Today, only 13 percent of all kids walk or bike to school.

Some of this change is due to where we're living. More Americans and Canadians now live in suburbs and "exurbs" than ever before. Between 1970 and 2000, the percentage of Americans living in suburbs or exurbs grew from 38 percent to 50 percent. In the past fifty years, over 90 percent of growth in United States metropolitan areas has been in the suburbs, where everything is more spread out, more driving is required, and sidewalks are often missing.

Suburban and exurban living has its benefits, but physical activity isn't one of them. Suburban dwellers are on average six pounds heavier than those who live in cities. Researchers have also connected time spent driving with obesity—the odds of being obese increase 6 percent with each hour per day spent in the car.

But the move to suburbia doesn't completely explain the disappearance of kids walking and biking to and from school. It's true that a smaller percentage of kids live within one mile of school (21 percent today versus 34 percent a generation ago) or two miles of school (35 percent versus 52 percent a generation ago). But these reductions pale in comparison with the rapid decline of kids walking or biking to and from school. Some other force is in effect here.

THE GOOD INTENTIONS OF PROTECTIVE PARENTS

An often overlooked factor also relates to the onset of the information age. In 1980, many parents were satisfied to know that their eleven-year-old son or their eight-year-old daughter was somewhere on the block, playing in a friend's backyard, or the next street over playing in an impromptu game of street football, or at the park four blocks away. Millions of calories were burned. But any parent would agree that there's much less of this kind of unstructured, unscheduled play outdoors than there was a generation ago.

Today, our standard of parenting has changed. The idea of letting your daughter play with friends in the nearby playground, unsupervised, is now seen as unacceptably risky by many parents. Some of this fear stems from the news coverage focused on child abductions and the other terrible things that happen to children. We're bombarded with news about the sensational cases of Elizabeth Smart or Shawn Hornbeck and we think, "That could happen to my child."

But here's the surprising thing: There's no evidence to suggest the prevalence of such horrific crimes has actually increased in the past generation. The risk of violent crime against kids ages twelve to nineteen has actually *dropped* over the past thirty years.

You'd never know this from watching the news. Individual incidents are so sensationalized that they lead to days, even weeks, of frenzied media coverage, and our awareness of such incidents is amplified to the point that our perception of the risk is warped. This warped perception is an important contributor to a much more probable risk: the risk that our child will become an obese adult.

Parents still want their kids to be active and to have fun. But their desire to protect their children's physical safety while still providing them with opportunities to be active has created the need to schedule activity. So now we have soccer on Wednesdays and Saturdays. Dance on Thursdays. Piano on Mondays. Boy Scouts on Thursdays. Worthy activities all, but they have come to define "activity" for our children—at the expense of all the unscheduled, spontaneous physical play that we all had as kids. As a result, mother and daughter alike think it's okay for Jane to spend three hours on MySpace after returning home from dance class, because she's had her activity for the day.

An important point to consider in all of this is the wear and tear on the parents. All these scheduled events require not only a significant level of planning, but also pickups and drop-offs, which in turn limit the amount of scheduled activity any one child or family can support. Plus, these scheduled pursuits and the resulting schlepping eat into family mealtimes, increasing the likelihood of going out to dinner, getting takeout, or eating a prepackaged, prepared meal at home.

THE MISTAKEN BELIEF THAT WEIGHT LOSS IS EASY

The final environmental enemy, ironically, is those who purport to actually help us lose weight. We're talking about the marketers of diet pills, supplements, exercise equipment—pretty much any weight-loss product that you see on infomercials, as well as some of the more well-established weight-loss companies. You could also include pharmaceutical companies in this category—those that are touting the promise of amazing new fat-burning drugs on the horizon. While they all market different products and services, they largely convey the same message:

Weight loss is quick.
Weight loss is easy.
Weight loss is convenient.

We've actually heard kids talk about their campaigns to *put on* weight, in order to qualify for weight-reduction surgery. Fourteen-year-old Jarrett F., who lost eighty pounds on the Sierras Solution program, said, "The message we're getting from society is we should eat more. Medicine will fix anything. You don't have to do any work, just go ahead."

And when we don't lose weight, how do we feel? Usually we feel dumb, lazy, and culpable. *If it's so easy, how come I can't do it?*

Well, now you know that it simply isn't true. Your child is fighting an uphill battle against a range of serious biological forces, in an environment seemingly designed for weight gain.

Let's be honest, to ourselves and to our children. There may be no harder battle in your child's life. Hard, yes. Impossible? No way. Biology is not destiny. And we can outsmart our environment. We've seen hundreds of kids lose weight, keep it off, and change the course of their lives. Your child can do it as well.

Helping Your Child Understand

You've seen that biological factors create real and powerful resistance to weight loss for your child. You know now that it is not simply a question of willpower over the temptations of an extremely powerful environment.

And when you think about it, the biology of obesity makes a lot of sense. Why would so many people have so much difficulty maintaining weight losses if biological forces did not resist weight loss? Losing weight produces many positive rewards, but relatively brief lapses in concentration, such as sporadic binges or inconsistent exercising, are eagerly greeted by billions of extra fat cells. That's a lot of hungry sparrows to feed! These fat cells and other biological forces are always present, ready to pounce.

When we explained these biological realities to fifteen-year-old Lauren S. she became quite upset, stunned at the power of it all. She said, "I can't believe it! All of my life people, including doctors, told me that my body was basically normal, fat but normal. Now you're telling me that I'm biologically abnormal and that this biology is the main cause of my weight problem? Why did I have to live the last ten years thinking that I was so pathetic? It's not just me or my personality. I really have to live with something that's a physical force within me."

Lauren's laments are very legitimate and painful. So many years lost to blaming herself and her "lack of willpower." Her first step was to accept the powerful role that biology plays in creating and maintaining weight problems. Once she did, she could deflect some of the blame and shame away from her personality and self-esteem.

Your child has definite biological challenges to overcome, like every overweight and formerly overweight person. She doesn't have to overcome her "weak" and "pathetic" personality. She doesn't have to shift from an abnormal state of gluttony to a normal state of controlled eating. That would be much easier. Unfortunately, your weight controller must change from a relatively normal state of functioning with an unfortunate biology to a set of behaviors that must be considered super-normal or extraordinary. This exceptional effort is what makes weight control one of the most complex athletic challenges a person can face.

Developing the Athlete's Mind-set

What does it take to run a five-minute mile? Of the three hundred million people in America, only a few thousand people can do this, and most of them are on track teams. How about running twenty-six sub-five-minute miles in a row? Only about a hundred people in the world can do that, and they're the ones running the New York and Boston marathons and making a living at it.

Can you imagine what it takes—the training, the focus—to do this? How about running twenty miles per day in high-altitude climates, which is what most of these elite marathon runners do to train? What about hitting a baseball thrown toward your head at one hundred miles per hour by a really large man? Or, consider the training required for a tennis player to hit a serve 130 miles per hour into a small square ninety feet away.

Elite athletes are certainly born with physical gifts, but all of them have transformed their bodies to take advantage of their talents and realize these remarkable feats. Elite athletes have realized that, regardless of their natural talent, they need to work to perform at the highest level.

Weight controllers are very similar. They've been born with a specific set of biological traits that make them exceptional. Only their own extraordinary efforts to work against these natural traits will help them get the desired performance out of their bodies.

We all wish we could accomplish our goals with minimal work. Jesse G., fifteen, who lost ninety-two pounds on the Sierras Solution, put it best. "The tricky thing was that I didn't really want to lose the weight by working at it," he said. "I wanted the weight to be gone, but I didn't want to put in the effort to make it happen. I just wanted it to be instant—one, two, three, *pow*—and I would be done."

Like Jesse G., most elite athletes would also rather sit on the couch and munch chips or even just rest more often. But they don't allow themselves to give in to such tendencies. Athletes have to get up early and train or stay out late and train some more. They require coaching, encouragement, knowledge of their sports, and the drive to keep at it even when the payoff isn't very apparent. They keep going because they trust the process. They know in their heart of hearts that they can do it, even when their bodies cry out for rest and relaxation. As your child goes through the program, you'll work together to develop the Athlete's Mind-set:

My extraordinary body demands
extraordinary efforts to create extraordinary results.

Become Your Child's Most Loyal Fan

When your child succeeds as a weight controller, he or she deserves the same credit and admiration that society gives successful athletes. Everyone understands how tough it is to run a four-minute mile; few have any real appreciation for the tenacity it takes to prevail over a weight-loss–resistant biology. When your child falters, and she will, she deserves sympathy or at least acceptance. She needs help and encouragement to try again soon, and to keep trying.

The most loyal fans might get disappointed by a loss, but they're in it for the long haul. Even if their team wins the championship this season, those fans know their team will have to fight just as hard again next year. Loyal fans don't ever give up; they just keep showing up to games and cheering their hearts out, year after year. Be the best, most loyal fan you can be, and your child will certainly make you proud.

PART 2

Creating the Sierras Solution Environment in Your Home

Chapter 3

Nurture the Desire to Change: Your Role as Weight-Control Coach

Newton's first law of physics is inertia. Inertia means that objects don't move unless they're forced to move. People are very much the same—we resist change mightily.

In their book *Facilitating Treatment Adherence*, Canadian psychologists Don Meichenbaum and Dennis Turk describe a remarkable example of how people resist change, despite sometimes dire consequences. Patients who were diagnosed with glaucoma—a serious but treatable eye disease—were told that they must use eyedrops three times per day or they would go blind.

The study revealed that only 42 percent of patients used the eyedrops as instructed. Remarkably, most failed to follow the regimen carefully enough to avoid permanent damage to their eyes. And even after becoming legally blind in one eye, only 28 percent changed course and began following the instructions more carefully.

These statistics are startling—and not at all uncommon. The fact is, people often struggle to maintain regimens of any kind that force them to behave differently from their usual routines.

As a parent, you can help your child work through some of the natural resistance to change. One of the best ways to start that is to empathize

> *If I got into a fight with my parents or something and they would go out to dinner, the second they walked out the door, I became a scavenger looking for something to eat. I'd look for a spoon and a jar of peanut butter and the whipped cream and anything and everything. Even if I wasn't mad at them, I'd be, like, "Oh well, they're not hounding me right now. I can shove everything in my mouth."*
>
> —LAUREN S., FIFTEEN,
> CALABASAS, CALIFORNIA
> INITIAL WEIGHT LOSS:
> FIFTY POUNDS IN FOUR MONTHS
> SUSTAINED WEIGHT LOSS:
> SIXTY-FOUR POUNDS AFTER ONE YEAR

and to let your child know that his or her experience is not unique; all personal change, whether simply adding a few daily drops to your eyes, or valiantly dropping a few dozen pounds, can be very challenging.

In this chapter, you'll learn how you can create the supportive and encouraging Sierras Solution environment in your home. Throughout the chapter, you'll notice how we emphasize how your positive reactions—to all feelings, changes, and successes or slipups—are essential to the Sierras Solution plan. Your unwavering support of and adherence to the plan are among the most important determining factors of your child's success. By the end of this chapter, you and your child will both have a clear picture of your mutual motivation to change, as well as your commitment to each other to make it happen.

Creating
the
Sierras
Solution
Environment
in
Your
Home

38

Nurture the Desire to Change

One of the major obstacles to establishing a desire to change is that many overweight children, teens, and young adults don't believe that anything can help them succeed. They have tried diet after diet, losing some weight, regaining it, and then gaining more. Most overweight kids have spent the better part of their lives failing at this, and the result is often resistance—sometimes fierce resistance—to change.

When you've discussed weight-loss programs with your child in the past, you've likely heard "Not me" and "I don't need to change." You may have responded with well-meaning pep talks or proposals to try a new diet or weight-loss scheme. He might have responded with a grimace, some folded arms, and maybe a slammed door. Discussion over.

Not this time. Your opening conversation will be your first moment on the Sierras Solution program.

OPENING THE CONVERSATION

Start off by making an appointment with your child. Tell him you have something very important you'd like to discuss with him, and you want the two of you to have uninterrupted time. Pick a time and day when you know he won't be tempted by the phone, a friend's visit, or a favorite TV show.

When you're sitting together—someplace comfortable, like the couch—turn to him and say, "Honey, I wonder how you're feeling about your weight these days. I know we've dealt with this in the past in different ways. How are you feeling about it right now?"

As your child responds, pay close attention. Really listen. Listen actively, letting your child know that you hear not only the specific words but the feelings behind them. Just sit and focus and tune in to him. For example:

> *Mom:* Let's talk about how you're feeling about your weight these days.
>
> *Bob* (fifteen years old): You know I hate to talk about this.
>
> *Mom:* I understand how frustrating it has been for you. I have some new ideas that really could make a difference for you, and for me—and us. But, first, I'd really like to know where you're at now. Tell me what you hate about talking about this, for example.
>
> *Bob:* I just hate being overweight and that I can't fix it. So few of my friends even think about their weight and I have to think about it, a lot.
>
> *Mom:* Yeah, I can see how unfair that must feel, especially when you watch Joe eat the universe and never gain any weight.

Without rushing, when the time seems right in this conversation, tell him about this book and a few things you've learned about the biology of weight loss.

If and when he's interested in hearing more, grab two notebooks, so you and your child can record some of your individual reactions during the rest of the discussion (or a later discussion, if you've agreed to let him think about it first). In these notebooks, you'll capture any initial thoughts and feelings and use them to craft your mutual goals for the program. We've found one of the most powerful ways to nurture the desire for change is to talk openly, sometimes for the first time, about the downsides of excess weight and the benefits of weight loss.

HELP YOUR CHILD ACKNOWLEDGE THE EMOTIONAL COST OF EXCESS WEIGHT

Perhaps you recall from chapter 1 that kids tend to view their overweight peers as "lazy, lying, cheating, sloppy, dirty, ugly, and stupid." While researchers have replicated these findings for more than forty years, you might be astonished to know that these words came from a study in which the participants were only *six years old*. The pain starts early, and it is fierce.

A recent study found that college students considered cocaine users, embezzlers, shoplifters, and blind people more suitable as potential marriage partners than obese people. A study at the University of Minnesota found that 96 percent of overweight adolescent girls reported incidents of verbal abuse. Another study found that 16 percent of employers said they wouldn't hire an overweight person under any condition. Every stage of the employment process shows strong biases against overweight people: selection, placement, compensation, promotion, discipline, and discharge. Unfortunately, even health-care workers, including physicians, show similar prejudices.

We know that kids vary in their sensitivity to such ugly behavior. But nearly 100 percent of AOS students have reported that excess weight creates an enormous emotional burden on them and that they have considerable difficulties managing these challenges. Low self-esteem, depression, irritability, insecurity, shyness, isolation, and anger are all very common consequences for overweight kids.

When we discuss these prejudices against overweight people with our students, they react with resentment and anger. Sharing this information about such bias with your weight controller may be difficult, but we believe it's not a bad idea. He might find it comforting to know that his experience is not unique and that he's not alone in this struggle. And seeing the downsides of his long-term prospects might also help generate some useful en-

Creating
the
Sierras
Solution
Environment
in
Your
Home

—

40

ergy. Fifteen-year-old Josh S., who has maintained a fifty-seven-pound weight loss for over a year, did an experiment to document the power of this prejudice in his own life.

> My best friend at military school and I were both on the football team and I hurt my leg. I could barely walk. Everyone said I was faking it because I was fat. I couldn't practice because I could barely walk. No one believed me and they all thought I was a wussy and all that stuff. So we did an experiment and we had my best friend pretend that his leg was hurt. Everyone believed him and felt sorry for him.

AOS students talk a lot about trying to get laws to ban this type of discrimination, similar to the laws against discrimination because of gender, race, religion, and age. We wish this were realistic, just as we wish that governments would take action and legislate and regulate away all the factors contributing to the obesity epidemic itself. What's more productive is to help your child channel this anger and resentment in healthy ways.

During your initial conversation, if your child seems up to it, talk about some of the research findings here. Ask your child, "How does it make you feel to hear that so many employers wouldn't hire someone, even if that person was great for the job, just because of his or her weight?" And ask, "What about the finding that ninety-six percent of overweight girls reported verbal abuse based on their weight?"

Again, listen to his response without judgment. Your child is probably as angry and resentful as Josh was. After listening to his feelings, try asking: "Now what, honey? What are you going to do about it?"

While one approach is to rail against the injustice of it all—and he most likely will, justifiably—try to use these emotions to help motivate him to return to a normal weight. Say, "Do you think we could try to get laws passed to ban this kind of ugly discrimination based on weight? What do you think of working toward that? What else could you do about these prejudices and abuse toward overweight people—something more personal? Do you think it works better to try to change the world on something like this or change yourself? Could you do both?"

Encourage your child to consider Josh's example. Josh took his ire and used it to help him become an expert in the Sierras Solution. He's now at a healthy weight and a successful LTWC.

Help Your Child Realize the Life-Changing Benefits of Weight Loss

Listen to some of the comments from kids who've used the Sierras Solution when they talk about what losing weight has done for them.

- "I just feel better about my appearance, so I'm more confident, and I'm more open to talking to more people and making friends."
- "I've gotten a lot of compliments on my changes. I'm now able to do more things that I couldn't do physically because I was overweight."
- "Now I like to run. I can climb things. I can do all that stuff that I couldn't do when I was a kid."
- "There is no doubt that people treat you better thin rather than overweight (unfortunately)."
- "Shopping is way easier. It's not even an issue now. I like to go shopping."
- "When I was overweight, I hated it. [Being at a normal weight is] a different lifestyle. It's like two different worlds."

Research shows that people who lose weight can experience major improvements in health, even by losing 5 to 10 percent of their initial weight. This 10 percent weight reduction has been linked to more balanced blood glucose, significantly lowered blood pressure, and lower cholesterol in the blood. In older people, losing twenty pounds can cut the risk of breast cancer by almost 20 percent—and even ten pounds lost decreased the chance of developing a host of other cancers. Not surprisingly, given these connections between modest weight loss and improvements in health risks, these relatively small weight losses could add multiple years to people's lives.

For young people, weight loss often leads to dramatic, clinically significant improvements in mood, including decreased risk for one of the major killers of young people—suicide. LTWCs enjoy increased social activities and improvements in satisfaction with personal relationships. We've also seen meaningful improvements in academic functioning follow considerable weight loss. One seventeen-year-old AOS student completed two years of high school work in nine months, as did several other younger students who had been struggling in school.

During your talk with your child, try to get him to imagine, in as much detail as possible, what it will feel like to be thinner. Ask him:

Creating
the
Sierras
Solution
Environment
in
Your
Home

42

- What would you do as a thinner person that you wouldn't do now?
- How would you feel when you got dressed in the morning?
- Would you have more confidence when you had something to say in class or just in talking to friends?
- How would you feel about meeting new people as a thin version of yourself?
- Would you feel better about yourself in sports or the gym or when you went swimming?

Please note: It's vitally important that you do all you can to help your child claim that new, thinner image of himself as the "true" him. Experts say that childhood and adolescence is a critical period in a person's emotional development, and researchers at the University of Pennsylvania have found that body images seem to crystallize during this time. Sadly, some weight controllers continue to feel negative about their bodies, regardless of the weight reduction (a fate not suffered by those who gain weight as adults). Don't let this window close while your child still thinks of himself as fat. By acting now, you could change the way he'll view himself for the rest of his life. (See "Building a Strong Body Image" on the next page for suggestions on how you can help your child develop a strong body image, starting today.)

HELP YOUR CHILD DETERMINE A PRIMARY MOTIVATION

How committed is your child to losing weight right now? Is it one of the top two or three life priorities at the moment? Or does it fall somewhere much farther down the list? Is it even on the list?

When overweight kids are not interested in losing weight, and are even hostile to the idea, we call this the Shock and Ambivalence phase of weight control. We'll talk about this and the other stages of weight loss more in chapter 4. If this is the case with your child, please consider enlisting some extra help. Turn to page 59 for our recommendations.

If your child agrees that she'd like to face the problem, but she feels deservedly gun-shy from her prior experiences, it's time to do what we call a Decision Balance Sheet. The principle is this: When you thoroughly analyze the possible advantages and disadvantages of a particular goal, you almost always become more committed to that goal. So by analyzing the

Building a Strong Body Image

Helping your child develop a positive body image is a lifelong gift. This technique can be a good start. First, create a two-column chart. Label one column with your name (or Mom, Dad) and the other with your child's name. Put the date on the top and a title such as "Good Stuff" or "Positive Features." Ask your child to stand in front of the mirror with you, starting first with a mirror that only reflects your faces. (Later you can do this exercise in front of a full-length mirror.)

As you look together, tell your weight controller what a lot of people your age would think to themselves as they look at themselves in a mirror: "Look at those wrinkles! You're getting so old! And look at that hair. It is just so much thinner and less full than it used to be." (You'll probably laugh together, which is good! It will help her to see that being so hard on yourself is a bit silly.) Then say, "Okay, let's see if both of us can find some things that we like about our physical selves. If we can focus on these things, we'll just feel better, stronger, and more confident."

Identify one thing about your face or hair that you like. Ask your child to do the same with herself. This could be a smile, a certain look in the eyes, skin tone or color, cheekbones, dimples, or any other feature. Write in a one- or two-word description in each of your columns. Repeat this with one or two more features.

Pick another physical aspect of yourself that you like, such as "strong legs," "energetic," or "good dancer." What physical things can your child do well? Encourage her to identify those strengths and write down at least one.

Talk about every sport both of you have tried and anything else that has a physical quality to it (such as good balance, bowling, swimming, holding breath underwater, endurance, even handwriting). Enter those items in your respective columns.

Leave a few lines at the bottom of each column and hang up the paper someplace in your house where you'll both see it regularly. Agree to add extra entries as they occur to you over the next week or so.

Talk about how it made both of you feel to complete this exercise. Did you both laugh and get into a good mood? Great—you obviously enjoyed naming the positive attributes of your physical selves. Urge your child (and yourself) to remember and focus on these positive attributes often. With a positive body image, you *both* can feel better about yourselves, all the time.

possible advantages and disadvantages of pursuing long-term weight control, your child is much more likely to commit to trying the Sierras Solution.

CREATE A DECISION BALANCE SHEET

We've compiled the example below of a Decision Balance Sheet from many children's responses. A blank form is included in Appendix 2. Please make a photocopy for your own use as well as your weight controller's, as you'll be revisiting and refining this document again and again.

Here's how to use this powerful tool.

Select a Goal

First, have your weight controller select a specific goal for the next year. For example, is your weight controller trying to lose twenty, or fifty, or one hundred pounds during this next year? When writing out the goal, consider that it works best to state a goal that is difficult but achievable. (See more on the importance and power of goals in chapter 4.) Outside of an immersion program like AOS, it is extremely difficult for anybody to lose one hundred pounds in one year regardless of the methods used. For most of us, a realistic goal for weight loss at home is between one-quarter to one pound per week. If your child is still growing, maintaining his or her current weight might also be a good goal.

If you and your child don't know what seems reasonable as a goal for weight loss, first calculate your child's body mass index (BMI). To do this, you can use the Baylor College of Medicine BMI calculator from a link at www.campwellspring.com/assessment.html. Just plug in your child's gender, age, height, and weight. After you click the "calculate" button, you'll see a BMI and a BMI percentile in the boxes at the bottom of the graph. Recalculate the BMI and BMI percentile by simply changing the weight. Try entering a weight that is twenty or thirty pounds less than your child's current weight. Watch the red dot move down until it's at the 85th level or below; that's a healthy weight range and a good weight goal. If the ultimate weight goal is a forty-pound weight reduction, a realistic goal for the next year might be a twenty-pound weight loss—truly a remarkable first step for one year. (If you want to do this calculation by hand, please see Appendix 6, Calculating Body Mass Index.)

Decision Balance Sheet: (EXAMPLE)

Name: Jane   Date: 3/3

What I'm trying to change this year: To lose twenty pounds

Importance Ratings: 10 = extremely important; 1 = not at all important

GOOD THINGS ABOUT DOING THIS	IMPORTANCE	CHALLENGING THINGS ABOUT DOING THIS	IMPORTANCE
Look better	10	I'll feel like a failure if I don't do it.	4
Feel better about myself sometimes	8	It will be frustrating sometimes.	7
Get new clothes	7	Maybe I still won't look too good.	3
Get cuter clothes	4	It will be hard work.	5
Fewer nasty comments	10	I might miss some foods.	7
Look more attractive to guys	7	Doing it will draw attention to me.	4
Healthier	4	I'll get tired.	4
Parents will be very proud	9		

Now create a goal for yourself to include on your own Decision Balance Sheet. To calculate your own BMI, either use the formula in Appendix 6 or search Google for "BMI calculator." For adults, a BMI over 30 is considered obese and a BMI between 25 and 29.9 is viewed as overweight. This wouldn't apply if you had greater muscle development than average people (virtually all NFL football players would be considered at least overweight, most obese, using this standard). You could set your own weight loss goals accordingly if your BMI and judgment indicate that you're overweight.

If you don't need to lose weight, perhaps you'll select "Run a 10K" or "Lower my cholesterol by 25 points." The point is that you will support your child's efforts by working alongside her on a challenging but achievable health and fitness goal for yourself. You show your willingness to put your behavior where your mouth is—you'll be "walking the walk."

Write Out the Pros and Cons

After you've both stated your goals, help each other write down everything you can think of that would be good or positive about reaching these goals. How would a twenty-pound weight loss affect your weight controller? How would a new fitness habit help you? Some parents of weight controllers have cited better relationships with their kids, less tension, easier socializing, more energy, and more confidence as examples of benefits.

After you've written down the good things, consider the challenges. Weight control takes time, effort, and money for everyone who seeks it. What are the specific costs of having your weight controller attempt to lose weight this year? Of pursuing your own health goals? Spend a few minutes writing out the challenges as well.

If you are seeking additional ideas, see whether discussing each item on the sample above would help generate additional points for your sheets. The more factors you can include on both sides, the better.

Review and Rate Each Entry

Review both columns carefully. Which column is more compelling? It's not a simple count of pros versus cons. This exercise requires you both to study the importance of each item on the lists. Take a few minutes to rate the importance of each item. Use a ten-point scale in which ten means "extremely important" and one means "not at all important." Some parents and kids find it fun and revealing to do this independently, and then swap papers.

In the sample above, you can see that Jane's challenges seem rather minor in most cases. For example, getting tired and feeling frustrated are temporary states and probably warrant low ratings. Also, you could make the point—in a kind and gentle way—that feeling a little tired or frustrated sometimes pales in comparison to feeling so much better physically and emotionally.

Balance Your Responses

Review your ratings and discuss them. See if you can come to some consensus about how to rate every item. If not, average your ratings, then put the average rating next to each item. Add up both columns.

In most cases, the column for the good things clearly outweighs the challenges. If this isn't the case, you might have to do a bit more work before your child is ready to start the Sierras Solution program.

The Decision Balance Sheet should remain an active part of the weight-control process. Please keep it handy and make copies so you can review it over and over again. Another option is to re-rate both columns, which weight controllers often find very motivating. This technique is particularly useful when the going gets a bit rough, such as when your child works hard but gains half a pound in a week. Keep your energy up and stay positive.

Keep It Positive

Creating
the
Sierras
Solution
Environment
in
Your
Home

48

Late-nineteenth-century physicians used lizard blood, crocodile dung, pig teeth, and frog sperm to "cure" their patients—and these approaches worked! Of course, these "treatments" didn't actually cure anything. Instead, medicine had tapped into the remarkable power of their patients' positive expectations.

Expectations are beliefs about what will happen. Consider what you and your weight controller could do if you could harness the power of positive expectations for good. After making an initial commitment to change, your beliefs about what you can and will change can keep you going or completely derail you. In the simplest terms:

The Power of Expectations

Mind over Muscle

Twenty-four men were tested for arm strength. Subjects were then paired and asked to arm wrestle each other. The researchers arranged the pairs so that one man was clearly stronger than the other. Incorrect information was deliberately provided to both wrestlers, so that both opponents expected the objectively weaker man to win. In other words, before actually wrestling, both men believed that the weaker man was actually the stronger man. Ten of the twelve contests (83 percent) were won by the man who had tested weaker! These results suggest that expectations can even overcome physical strength.

If you expect to succeed, you really might.
If you expect to fail, you probably won't succeed.

Psychologists have studied the power of positive thinking for more than sixty years. While positive belief about success cannot in and of itself get your weight controller to walk an hour a day or order fruit instead of cheesecake, optimism works much better than pessimism.

Perhaps you've heard the old schoolteacher's adage, "Catch them being good." Compliments, positive attention, encouragement, and tangible rewards definitely help maintain motivation. Try to convey an appreciation for the challenges that your weight controller is facing with every opportunity. If you can do this, and remain optimistic about your child's capabilities, you will go a long way toward keeping your child motivated to stay on track.

CUE INSTEAD OF NAG

We sincerely doubt that a single parent has ever roamed the earth without doing some nagging. Watching your children cause themselves harm elicits incredibly powerful emotions. All parents naturally aim to get their children to take good care of themselves and to do things in constructive,

We tried absolutely everything. We used threats, bribes, and cajoling. And we said things like, "If you keep eating, this is what's going to happen . . ." We used scare tactics and everything else we can think of. We tried absolutely every diet and every strategy. Nothing worked. What do you do? So, I withdrew. I said to myself, "It must be me. I must be causing the problem," and I shut up. It didn't get any better.

We were so frustrated for so many years, we wound up nagging instead of letting Jessie take responsibility for his own thing. We were taking responsibility. So, in essence, I had to learn to give up that responsibility and give him ownership of his own weight.

—AUDREY G., JESSE G.'S MOTHER
JESSE'S INITIAL WEIGHT LOSS: EIGHTY-EIGHT POUNDS IN SIX MONTHS
JESSE'S SUSTAINED WEIGHT LOSS: NINETY-TWO POUNDS AFTER SIX ADDITIONAL MONTHS

not destructive, ways. This typically involves nagging, which is a common and miserable part of the lives of weight controllers and their parents.

Instead of nagging, we recommend cueing. Cues are words that stimulate or suggest appropriate actions, without insisting on those actions.

In order to even consider this strategy, parents must accept one unavoidable fact: you cannot nag your child into successful weight control. The research supports this conclusion. One recent survey of nine-year-olds showed that about 50 percent spent their own money on snacks and other foods over a two-week period. If nine-year-olds are buying food outside of the home, virtually all teens have or can find the resources to do so. As parents today, you must accept that your young weight controller is the captain of his or her fate in this regard. If you nag and cajole and argue, you'll only put a greater distance between you and your young weight controller.

To understand the distinction between cueing and nagging, consider the following situation, taken from the lives of one of our students about two months after he left AOS. The father has a tendency to work long hours, to promise to come home for dinner, and then fail to show up as promised. The son has developed considerable resentment and anger about this.

On this day, the father promised to be home by 7:00 to have dinner with

Creating
the
Sierras
Solution
Environment
in
Your
Home

50

his son and wife. Very soon after the son and his mother had eaten dinner, the son grabbed a large bag of low-fat potato chips and dumped it into a big mixing bowl. He was watching a movie in the living room when his father finally showed up, about an hour later than promised. (As you read, think about how you would handle this situation.)

> Father: Hey, how are you doing?
> Son: I'm okay, I guess.
> Father: I'm really sorry that I'm late again. I just couldn't get away on time.
> Son: Yeah.
> Father: Didn't you just have dinner?
> Son: Yeah, so what?
> Father: Well, I don't get why you're eating a giant bowl of potato chips right after eating dinner. That doesn't seem like part of the Sierras Solution.
> Son: Screw you, Dad! (Son storms out of the room and slams the door to his room.)

What happened here? An angry teenager reacted to his father after his father tried using nagging to encourage his son to reduce overeating. Nagging usually doesn't work, but can prove especially volatile when feelings of anger are bubbling up in the teenager at the time the parent starts to nag.

Consider an alternative, which we call "cueing," applied in the same scenario:

> Father: Hey, how you doing?
> Son: Okay, I guess.
> Father: Sorry I'm late again. I just couldn't get away.
> Son: Yeah.
> Father: I can see you're probably pissed off at me and I can understand that.
> Son: Yeah, I really wish you would get home when you said you would.
> Father: I am very sorry and you're right. I really have to concentrate on that, especially when I make a specific promise.
>   I'm noticing the bowl of potato chips and I assume you've just finished eating dinner. I know this is your program, but I just wanted to

My parents and I used to have this dynamic where I thought they were trying to control me. And they thought I was doing it to spite them. Both of those points were true sometimes. Now if they're upset or if they're worried about my program, they'll say, "Just make sure you're self-monitoring," and I'll say, "Thank you," and we'll be done with it. There's none of this passive-aggressive, we're-resentful-of-each-other thing. It's just really straightforward and honest.

—LINDSAY S., SEVENTEEN, PALO ALTO, CALIFORNIA
    INITIAL WEIGHT LOSS: SEVENTY-FOUR POUNDS IN TWELVE MONTHS
    SUSTAINED WEIGHT LOSS: EIGHTY POUNDS AFTER ONE MONTH

mention that if you wanted to talk about something, anything, I'm here for the rest of the night.

Son: Yeah, it is my program and my bowl of potato chips. I don't want to talk right now, but I'll keep that in mind.

You can see many differences in the outcome when using this cueing procedure instead of nagging. The son didn't storm off and didn't explode with additional anger. He may or may not have stopped eating his bowl of potato chips. He may or may not have taken his father's invitation to talk. However, by handling the situation this way, the father can help the son see the link between his current eating behavior and his long-term goals. At least this cue has a chance of changing his son's behavior—if not immediately, then possibly later that evening or the next day. Nagging has virtually no chance of success, and may have some unpleasant and potentially damaging consequences for the relationship.

Try discussing this type of cueing openly and honestly with your young weight controller. You can let him or her know that you plan to do this when you see instances of problematic eating. You will recognize what he's doing and simply describe it in simple terms without invoking any negativity or criticism, if at all possible. Tone tends to communicate more than words; it helps if you bear this in mind.

Creating
the
Sierras
Solution
Environment
in
Your
Home

52

Minimize Negative Comments, Including Teasing

This one is obvious. However, siblings or friends of siblings often make remarks that are quite negative and hurtful. Sometimes parents do this, too, without meaning to. Some overweight kids have gotten used to such barbs and have learned to laugh them off. But for most, these comments eat away at them and generally make them miserable.

Agree to a family ban. Having the family agree to limit any kind of teasing or offhand remarks or "little jokes" along these lines can help a weight controller feel more positive and motivated.

Encourage everyone to enforce the ban. Explicitly instruct all family members to police this agreement, even with those who are invited into the house.

Talk with your child about how to handle such comments. Together, develop an arsenal of responses. Probably the best thing your weight controller can do is to walk away whenever possible. Craft a standby retort, such as "I don't think it's funny to make a joke at my expense, especially when you know how hard I work at this." Or "That's not at all funny to me." These assertive statements let the teaser know that such comments are not humorous—they're hurtful.

Encourage Positive Self-Support Techniques

Help him create a number of positive self-support techniques that will reinforce his motivation to change.

Encourage Your Child to Find Motivating Images

Suggest that your child carry a picture of herself at either slimmer or heavier weights to motivate her, or find other motivating images in magazines. Some weight controllers like to hang pictures or posters of activities like rafting or tennis, or even photos of clothes, to keep them focused. If your child is keen on fitting into an old outfit, consider hanging the outfit where it can be seen. Concentration boils down to thinking about something quite often. Images help weight controllers remember their goals.

Teach "Premacking"

This technique will positively reinforce your LTWC's commitment. "Premacking" (named for psychologist Dr. David Premack) involves rein-

Sierras Solution Success Story—Dan K

Dan K. arrived at AOS depressed and feeling hopeless about the future. Although he did quite well in school, he was socially isolated—he had few friends and spent most of his time playing video games and reading. As he lost his weight, Dan transformed into a showstopping musical performer and one of the school's most popular students.

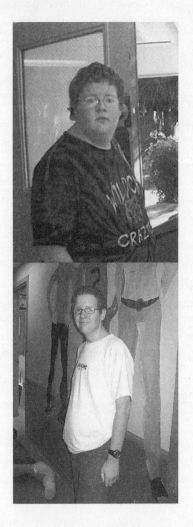

For as long as I can remember, I've always had a weight problem. Since kindergarten, I would be playing games with friends and finding out (often painfully and embarrassingly) that I couldn't do everything they could. When older kids would call me names, the others would join in. I would often cry and scream.

You might think that as the kids around me grew older, they'd learn that they were truly hurting me and lay off. But as my peers grew older, their ridicule and cruelty got worse and worse. By eighth grade, I was a pessimistic 287-pound ball of misery and hate. I hated school, I hated life, but, above all, I hated myself. I began having thoughts of suicide. Thanks to friends, family, and a good therapist, I saw what I had become, and I promised myself I'd never, ever let myself get that low ever again.

As I entered high school, I was still a 290-pound wreck. Then my mom heard about AOS. After going through the program, I can no longer call myself a 290-pound emotional wreck. Hell, I can't even call myself a wreck! Though I'm still somewhat insecure and unhappy at times, it's far from the

(continued)

old me who would write all over his desk about how much he hated it all. For the first time in my life, I am happy and I love myself. I can run, jump, and do things that everyone else can. I know I am not worthless or inferior. I have improved by leaps and bounds, and I continue to improve day by day. I'm not yet sure what the future holds, but I plan on facing it head-on, full of enthusiasm.

—Dan K., fifteen, Omaha, Nebraska
   Initial weight loss: 129 pounds in nine months
   Sustained weight loss: 128 pounds for ten months

forcing an unlikely behavior by pairing it with a likely behavior. In this example, have your LTWC write down several key words on half of an index card and have him place the card in his wallet. Here's what he might write:

- Acceptance
- Self-esteem
- Mastery
- Clothes
- Health
- Energy
- Looks

Left to his own devices, reviewing these words regularly would be an "unlikely behavior" for him. But with Premacking, every time he uses his wallet (a common or "very likely" behavior), he will take a few seconds to review the card, remember the value of feeling more energetic and looking good, get those positive expectations flowing more intensely, and renew his commitment to weight control.

Even in the most positive and supportive of families and households, every single weight controller will experience setbacks. In fact, their setbacks will likely follow a very specific pattern. Knowing what to expect can help both of you persevere.

Chapter 4

Navigate the Six Stages of Change: Guide Your Child Through the Predictable Pattern of Weight Loss

Right now, what do you expect to experience on the Sierras Solution program? How will you feel when you watch and participate in your child's efforts at weight control? What does your weight controller expect? If you don't know the answers, ask yourself and your child, "What will this experience be like, on a daily, weekly, monthly, and yearly basis?"

Some kids expect to struggle and resent the process; others expect to change and look forward to it. Young weight controllers struggle more than adults with staying on track when they are frustrated. The road to successful weight control is bumpy—usually very bumpy. When kids and parents understand the nature of the bumps, they can better anticipate and cope with them.

As you go along in the program, you may come to a phase when you think your child needs some help with motivation, and she probably does. But it could also be that she's simply going through a natural stage in her evolution as an LTWC.

Researchers have identified three primary and three secondary stages of change in long-term weight control. The vast majority of weight controllers will experience the primary stages: honeymoon, frustration, and acceptance. Only a relatively small proportion of weight controllers seem to ex-

Stages of Change in Successful Weight Control

PRIMARY STAGES

HONEYMOON → FRUSTRATION ↔ ACCEPTANCE

SECONDARY STAGES

Shock/Ambivalence   Fear of Success   Lifestyle Change

Based on Kirschenbaum, D. S., et al. 1992. Stages of change in successful weight control: A clinically derived model. *Behavior Therapy* 23:623–635.

perience one or more of the secondary stages: shock/ambivalence, fear of success, and lifestyle change.

As you review the descriptions of these stages, see if you can tell which stage best captures where your weight controller is at the moment and where she has been over the past couple of years. The three primary stages of weight control describe the process of weight control over a long period of time.

Sometimes things go well. Other times the struggle is hard to tolerate. The double-headed arrow in the illustration demonstrates that there is movement back and forth between the frustration and acceptance stages. The world never stops being frustrating, so your weight controller will probably face frustration many times. But after a while, every successful weight controller gets to acceptance and truly becomes an LTWC.

Primary Stage 1: Honeymoon

I was just so happy. And the weight was just coming off so fast. And I lost thirty pounds my first month. And I just wanted to do everything.

—Josh S., fifteen, Tucson, Arizona
  Initial weight loss: sixty-two pounds in five months
  Sustained weight loss: fifty-seven pounds for more than one year

Navigate the Six Stages of Change: Guide Your Child Through the Predictable Pattern of Weight Loss

Weight controllers in this initial stage often express delight, joy, and a sense of genuine satisfaction. They are relieved to find something that is helping to reduce the frustration and anger they feel about their weight. They eagerly embrace the new weight-control program, reflecting a strong commitment to change.

Honeymooners are very careful about doing each and every element of their weight-control program. They self-monitor consistently, and spend time reading about weight control and exercise. Honeymooners also talk enthusiastically with others about health, weight control, and related topics.

HOW YOU CAN HELP

The honeymoon stage may last several weeks, several months, or even a year. If your weight controller is at this stage, you'll have an easy time keeping your child interested and working hard, at least for a while.

Secondary Stage 1: Shock and Ambivalence

> When I was gaining the weight, I thought, "Well, if I just keep eating, I'll be big enough to get the surgery." My parents would tell me not to count on that surgery, but I always did. I remember thinking that everyone who went to AOS was probably a freak with lots of problems. I couldn't see that I needed to be there.
>
> —HENRY E., SIXTEEN, COLUMBUS, OHIO
>   INITIAL WEIGHT LOSS: 108 POUNDS IN SIX MONTHS
>   SUSTAINED WEIGHT LOSS: 108 POUNDS FOR OVER 1½ YEARS

Creating
the
Sierras
Solution
Environment
in
Your
Home

—

58

Some weight controllers react with surprise and even anger about the nature of the battle they must face with their own biology and culture. Most of us are used to getting what we want, when we want it. Weight control simply does not work that way. In this somewhat less common stage, some weight controllers become skeptical about the value of working so hard for so long. They seem disappointed and annoyed. "There must be an easier way of doing this!" is the key statement of the shock and ambivalence stage.

From the outside world's perspective, teenagers in this stage seem firmly planted in denial and defensiveness. This stage is not uncommon in the first few days of a new student's enrollment at AOS. We often hear statements like:

- *I really don't want to be here and don't need to be here.*
- *I could do this myself if my parents would just help me out more.*
- *I just don't see my weight as much of a problem.*

Weight controllers tend to jump from one approach to another during this stage. They may try a new diet, or join one health club or another, or try a weight-management program and then drop out. The quest for the quick fix characterizes this stage. Teens, many of whom struggle with authority anyway, may reject any suggestion from others and insist on doing it their own way.

How You Can Help

Shock and ambivalence create significant problems, but the best way to overcome them is to see that weight loss is possible. "When I got to AOS, I was, like, 'I'm not the problem. You're the problem,'" recalls Terry H. "But once the weight started to come off, I was jubilant."

If you find your weight controller resisting a lot, despite your best efforts, you will do well to consider adding structures that lead to success. (See "Provide Structure," on page 193.) There's no point in arguing with shock and ambivalence. If you can get your weight controller to a place where he can see that he can do it, his ambivalence will change to excitement.

Primary Stage 2: Frustration

I was just bored. I was tired of doing the same activities, but I didn't have the motivation to do anything new either, so I just didn't like doing activities.

—Brittany B., fifteen, Carpinteria, California
Initial weight loss: forty-seven pounds in five months
Sustained weight loss: fifty-nine pounds for almost one year

In this stage, weight controllers often think about going back to old patterns of eating and (in)activity. They seem to long for the old days. After all, the old ways are easier and take much less time and energy. When they're in frustration, weight controllers resent the effort required for successful weight control. They compare themselves to people who are not overweight and people who have never been overweight. This is a "why me?" stage. "Why do I have to work at this all the time?" "Why can't I take a break every once in a while?" "Why don't my skinny friends have to do this?" In this stage, weight controllers battle life's basic unfairness.

Weight controllers in the frustration stage become less careful about their eating and activity. They do not monitor their eating and exercising as well as they did in the honeymoon stage. They are much less attentive to most aspects of the program that they adhered to so well in the honeymoon stage. The expression "hanging in there" (sometimes just barely) describes frustration well.

How You Can Help

Unfortunately, the frustration stage can last quite a while—sometimes months—and prove very challenging to you when your weight controller gets there. Try some of the suggestions here to help your weight controller understand that these problems, distractions, and discouraging moments happen to *everybody*—absolutely every single weight controller. The key is persistence.

Shift Attitudes

Some weight controllers talk to themselves when they're struggling with frustration. They talk about the nature of their struggle and try to convince themselves to move closer to an acceptance of that challenge.

Change Expectations

Some weight controllers have an extremely tough biology that resists anything but the most modest weight loss. Weight loss may not happen every week and does not appropriately reflect the degree of effort involved. Ask your child what he expects to happen—does he expect to lose weight every week? If so, try to make it clear that the process of following the three Simple Changes counts far more than the outcome in any given week (see chapter 6).

Creating

the

Sierras

Solution

Environment

in

Your

Home

———

60

Get Back to Basics

When tennis players find their serves missing the mark, they look at fundamentals, like the positioning of their shoulders and the precise positioning of their hand on the racquet. Encourage your LTWC to focus on the fundamentals—staying under 20 grams of fat per day, taking at least ten thousand steps a day, and self-monitoring consistently—when he finds himself struggling. Or he could even focus on one particular goal, such as much more vigorous activity or an intense focus on fat grams and calories.

> *I have a hoodie that I used to fit into pretty well and now it's huge. I could fit two people in there. I keep it hanging on my door.*
>
> —JOSH S., FIFTEEN, TUCSON, ARIZONA
>   INITIAL WEIGHT LOSS: SIXTY-TWO POUNDS IN FIVE MONTHS
>   SUSTAINED WEIGHT LOSS: FIFTY-SEVEN POUNDS FOR ONE YEAR

Emphasize Activity

Encourage your weight controller to always clip on the pedometer—failing to hit the ten-thousand-step mark every day will cause the metabolism to slow down and the appetite to increase. (More on this in chapter 6.) Get your weight controller involved in fun new activities, like martial arts, bowling, squash, or racquetball, or any new sport. Even participating in a school play can break a cycle of relative inactivity.

Weight Loss Matters

Remember that the longer your weight controller can stay tough in the fight, and the closer your weight controller gets to a normal weight range, the easier it will become to break through frustration once and for all. Weight loss itself is often the key catalyst to reaching the acceptance stage. The difference in self-esteem, mood, attitude, outlook, and energy between an obese student and a student who has reached a normal weight range for the first time in memory is like night and day. And the latter tends to be able to shake off frustration more quickly and easily.

Navigate the Six Stages of Change: Guide Your Child Through the Predictable Pattern of Weight Loss

———

Secondary Stage 2: Fear of Success

I had established myself as overweight and didn't know myself any other way. So I was afraid to change, in a sense, because I was afraid that I wouldn't know myself.

—ALLISON G., TWENTY, WICHITA, KANSAS
INITIAL WEIGHT LOSS: SEVENTY-FIVE POUNDS IN SIX MONTHS
SUSTAINED WEIGHT LOSS: EIGHTY-FOUR POUNDS FOR SIX ADDITIONAL MONTHS

Occasionally, some weight controllers worry about succeeding. Although most people, including almost every teenager in the world, would love to become "too thin" or "too sexy," some actually worry about this. For the few who experience a genuine fear-of-success stage, the thought of these changes or compliments from others can produce anxiety and worry. Weight controllers in this stage may sabotage their own efforts. They might eat with people who usually consume high-fat foods. They might begin cooking and baking too much. They might put themselves in situations that produce too much eating or not enough activity.

HOW YOU CAN HELP

Fear of success is another stage that can create significant problems for weight controllers. This technique can help your weight controller if she seems afraid of losing weight.

Try Counterrationalization
In stark contrast to the strategy for getting over shock and ambivalence—not to argue at all—this strategy is a supremely logical form of argument. The first step is to identify the underlying assumptions. Ask your child, "What's your biggest fear about this process?" Then, using the chart that begins on the next page, get at the underlying distorted assumption and counter with some rational good sense. Your teenager might like this: an invitation to argue!

Help Your Child Create a Mental Marquee Message
Once you've worked with the counterrationalization exercise, encourage your child to create one powerful, versatile statement that will support her

Creating
the
Sierras
Solution
Environment
in
Your
Home

———

62

Fears	Assumptions	Counterrationalizations
I will gain back the weight that I have lost.	I am destined to fail.	Managing weight is a difficult task. Making mistakes is a part of any learning process. I am still learning to manage my weight; I can expect lapses from time to time. I can learn more about myself and successful weight management by learning from my lapses.
I am afraid others will see me fail if I gain the weight back.	I will be judged critically by others even when evidence does not warrant such judgments.	Not everyone is concerned about my weight. Many people can be sympathetic and respect how hard I am trying. Being overly concerned with others' opinions of me is a burden I give myself. I can choose to ignore what others say and appreciate what I learn about myself day to day.
I am worried that even if I lose all the weight, my body won't be the way I want it to be.	I will not get what I want from this process, so why should I try?	I don't need to be perfect in order to feel good about my many successes. I can accept the reality that my body is not perfect. I can feel proud of my efforts to manage my weight. I can find satisfaction in knowing that every moment of exercise and every pound of weight lost makes me stronger and healthier.

Fears	Assumptions	Counterrationalizations
I am afraid I won't like myself after I lose the weight.	I will not feel positive about the outcome of this process.	Making arbitrary negative predictions will not benefit me. I am much more than my weight. There are many things I like about myself.
I am afraid that if I spend more time exercising, I will feel like the dumb gym rats I never respected.	People who exercise frequently are overly focused on themselves and dumb.	I have an obese physiology that resists change. Frequent exercise is one way that I can take care of myself that seems good for me, not a sign of a big ego or stupidity.
If I lose more weight, I won't be able to use my weight as an excuse.	I believe that life is unmanageable without such excuses.	This is an opportunity to learn something about myself and to develop new and better ways of coping with the challenges that are before me.
I want to scream when people compliment me.	I feel that others are only concerned with my looks and not me as a person. I feel excessive pressure to maintain the loss when others notice my weight loss.	I cannot control the attitudes of others. Some people who offer compliments recognize and respect the hard work required to manage weight. I have worked hard to be successful with weight loss and deserve the praise that others offer. I do not have to think of their praise as a burden or pressure. I can decide how much to pressure myself to maintain the weight loss.
I am afraid someone might ask me for a date.	I must go on the date.	I can always say no.
I am afraid someone will see me and want to have sex.	I must have sex.	I can always say no.

Fears	Assumptions	Counterrationalizations
I am afraid others will respond to me because I am attractive and not because of who I am.	I believe that my behavior automatically results in specific judgments by others.	Being overly concerned with the opinions of others is a burden I give myself. My feelings about myself are more important than the opinions of others. People do respond to each other in part because of attractiveness. Those responses, however, will not determine my worth or character.

when she comes up against one of these fears. For example, "There is no conceivable way that the life which I am now leading would be worse than that which I endured when I weighed forty pounds more than I do now."

Primary Stage 3: Acceptance

I think that what changed the most was my attitude. Before, I was really depressed and I didn't really feel that great about myself. And now I feel like I can do pretty much anything as long as I try.

—HILLARY K., SEVENTEEN, SENECA, SOUTH CAROLINA
INITIAL WEIGHT LOSS: SIXTY POUNDS IN FIVE MONTHS
SUSTAINED WEIGHT LOSS: SIXTY-THREE POUNDS FOR OVER ONE YEAR

This is the stage when LTWCs settle in for the long haul. They experience a peaceful sense of resolve about weight control. They are comfortable; they have a clear sense that they can manage and overcome their challenging biology. They also refine their knowledge of nutrition. Their understanding of the factors that affect weight control is also clear. They still struggle with consistency of focus and commitment, particularly when they go on vacation or when illness or travel disrupts their schedule.

When weight controllers reach the acceptance stage, they have developed very consistent patterns of activity. They view activity as either enjoyable or at least acceptable. They no longer see it as drudgery but as something that can help them. So they maintain a positive and effective attitude toward it.

When they reach acceptance, weight controllers do not battle with themselves anymore. They also assert themselves effectively in restaurants and other social situations regarding food. For example, weight controllers in the acceptance stage would not accept a chicken entrée ordered "grilled, as dry as possible" if it's served swimming in butter. They would ask the server to have the dish prepared again. They do not feel deprived, frustrated, or very guilty when they ask a server to prepare their food in a healthful way. They feel taken care of and happier when they can get food prepared the way they now "prefer."

Can you really prefer baked potatoes to French fries? Fresh berries to chocolate mousse? Cheeseless pizza to cheese pizzas smothered in sausage or pepperoni? Some LTWCs might say, "No way! I'll eat the healthier alternatives almost all of the time, but no one can convince me that low-fat tastes better than high-fat. Get real!" But most in acceptance say, "Sure. That food tastes fine and just works better for my body."

HOW YOU CAN HELP

LTWCs in acceptance still struggle with certain situations and experience lapses in activity and eating—even occasional binges. Disruptions in routines can disrupt focus enough to create major challenges. When LTWCs are in school, for example, there are fewer opportunities to snack during the day—but during holidays and vacations, opportunities to snack and rationalize abound. You might hear an LTWC in acceptance say, "But I'm supposed to be on vacation." Or "We always stop at that doughnut place on this trip." Variations on the theme of "I deserve it" sometimes emerge.

Encourage Comparisons
Once your LTWC generally understands his compromised biology, help him to compare himself to others who are struggling. Successful LTWCs recognize that many people face much more difficult and unpleasant ways of living. Gently remind him that he has a very wide range of foods to

Creating
the
Sierras
Solution
Environment
in
Your
Home

——

66

choose from, many of which are quite satisfying and comforting, and encourage him to accept that particular range of food and learn to enjoy it.

Restate the Facts

LTWCs in the acceptance stage generally stay on track because they accept that "this is the way my body works."

Secondary Stage 3: Lifestyle Change

I exercise pretty much every day now. If I didn't ride my bike for a week, for example, I'd feel lazy. In fact, if I didn't do something for two days, I'd feel a strong urge to do something active.

—BRITTANY B., FIFTEEN, CARPINTERIA, CALIFORNIA
  INITIAL WEIGHT LOSS: FORTY-SEVEN POUNDS IN FIVE MONTHS
  SUSTAINED WEIGHT LOSS: FIFTY-NINE POUNDS FOR ALMOST ONE YEAR

This is the ultimate goal. LTWCs in this difficult-to-reach stage are very confident and aggressively self-protective. They are adamantly unwilling to return to a lifestyle where they were mindless about their eating, activity, and weight. They carefully observe their eating and activity. They are very aware of changes in their moods, routines, relationships, work, and anything else that might trigger poor food choices or overeating. They are confident about their knowledge of weight control—what works and what does not. Their eating and activity patterns are less tied to emotions than they used to be. They carefully monitor their eating and weight. They weigh themselves regularly even if they had a bad day or a bad week. When problems with eating or activities emerge, they view these lapses as challenges to be solved. They do not view problematic eating or lapses in their usual activity routines as weaknesses in their personalities or as reasons to give up.

As this stage requires a high level of maturity and judgment, relatively few teens are able to get here. Some do, usually after a couple of years of using the Sierras Solution. Most will do very well at the acceptance stage, but those LTWCs who get to lifestyle change are fairly set for life.

Navigate the Six Stages of Change: Guide Your Child Through the Predictable Pattern of Weight Loss

——

Sierras Solution Success Story—Jill R.

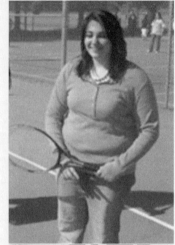

Jill remembers being overweight since preschool. She began dieting early on, and nothing seemed to work. Starting in seventh grade, a series of unhealthy decisions and disappointing friendships led to depression, which led to more weight gain. At AOS, one key part of Jill's success was the passion she developed for running. Though running was painful initially, it soon became a healthy coping skill. Her new motto is "I will grow on the inside as I shrink on the outside."

Weight has always been an issue in my life. I was active, but I ate really unhealthy. My weight started to become a major issue after my problems in seventh grade. I started to make the wrong choices with the people I hung out with and the things I was doing. I got suspended from my school. I was depressed and didn't know what to do with myself but eat my feelings away.

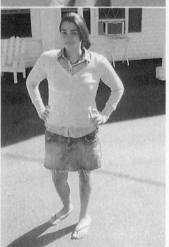

I never noticed how big I had actually become until one day I looked in the mirror and I realized I really needed to do something about it. It had taken over my life completely. I was also treated a lot differently from my family and friends. When my mom started to notice how much weight I was packing on, she got scared and so did I. I disappointed myself that I let it go that much and I knew I needed to do something about it. I had become extremely unhealthy emotionally and physically.

Now, I look back and realize that a year ago I weighed 230 pounds. I was in denial about the weight, depressed, hopeless, and couldn't run as much as a

(continued)

couple of feet. Six months after leaving AOS, I weigh eighty pounds less. I joined my school's cross-country team, which I love. Recently, I ran the Bay State Half Marathon and finished 792 out of 2,000. The first thought that popped into my head was—AOS. AOS truly saved my life. I couldn't be more thankful.

—JILL R., FOURTEEN, FITCHBURG, MASSACHUSETTS
   INITIAL WEIGHT LOSS: SEVENTY-SIX POUNDS IN NINE MONTHS
   SUSTAINED WEIGHT LOSS: EIGHTY POUNDS FOR MORE THAN SIX MONTHS

One of their strongest traits is that they've learned to handle stressful situations directly without using food as a coping mechanism. They enjoy eating and find eating calming and relaxing. They even eat more than they would like to occasionally. However, they almost never overeat high-fat foods. They also actively seek healthful eating and activity opportunities, even when their lives are disrupted by travel, vacations, demanding projects, or illness.

The mastery of stress-management skills not only helps your child maintain a healthy lifestyle, it is also a common trait among the most happy adults. Let's look at how you can help your child to develop these skills so she can follow her dreams more comfortably and happily.

Chapter 5

Help Your Child Manage Stress: Tips and Strategies for Overcoming Emotional Eating

I was at a high school pep rally with my entire freshman class. These two guys had cut out a newspaper clipping that had a picture of two really fat people, with captions saying, "Noticing your clothes don't fit anymore?" and "You know you're so fat when . . ." These boys had put my name on one of the pictures and they gave it to me in front of the whole entire freshman class. And they let me sit there and cry. I just remember going home and sitting there and eating and eating because I didn't know what else to do. I figured that's what my life is going to be like from now on.

—Vicki M., fourteen, Fairfax, Virginia
Initial weight loss: sixty-six pounds in six months
Sustained weight loss: fifty-four pounds for six additional months

Like Vicki M., most overweight kids at least occasionally use food as a coping mechanism to deal with unpleasant emotions. Using this response to stress frequently can make weight control extremely difficult. A recent study of 4,320 children by Drs. Martin Cartwright, Jane Wardle, and their colleagues from University College London showed that greater stress is associated with increased fatty-food intake, less fruit and vegetable intake, more snacking, and less eating of breakfast.

While overweight and nonoverweight children might both respond to stress in this way, the biology of overweight children is much less forgiving; the additional fat promotes the expansion of millions of fat cells. Often, the weight gain that results from frequent emotional eating itself becomes a source of stress, and the child finds herself trapped in an extremely vicious cycle.

Successful LTWCs learn how to handle challenging situations without resorting to self-destructive eating or decreasing their activity level. One of the most important things you can do as a parent is help your weight controller improve her stress management skills and deal with her emotions more effectively. The first step is to understand stress—where it comes from and how your child reacts to it.

> *My weight didn't become a major problem for me, in part because I have a lot of friends. There were people who taunted me and ridiculed me, especially in elementary school. But I had friends who stuck through it with me and I know they were with me not because of how I looked or what I have, but because they're my real friends.*
>
> —LAUREN E., FIFTEEN, HOUSTON, TEXAS
>   INITIAL WEIGHT LOSS: FORTY-SIX POUNDS IN FOUR MONTHS
>   SUSTAINED WEIGHT LOSS: FIFTY-TWO POUNDS FOR OVER ONE YEAR

The Difference Between Stress and Stressors

As you know from experience, not everyone reacts to challenging situations and circumstances in the same way. There are actually two parts of what we typically call "stress"—the challenging situation, and the reaction to the situation.

Stressors, such as the ridicule and teasing endured by Vicki M., are demands from others or from the environment. For many overweight kids, simply passing by a once-favored fast-food restaurant can be a stressor.

Help Your Child Manage Stress: Tips and Strategies for Overcoming Emotional Eating

—

Stress is the negative feelings a child could feel in response to those environmental demands or challenges. Stressors needn't cause stress. Consider the example of Lauren E. (see preceding page).

Lauren E. coped with the stressor of taunting by talking to her supportive friends; she never felt stress because she had a healthful coping mechanism that worked for her. But without using positive coping mechanisms, most kids will experience significant stress.

Stressors are generally unpredictable and/or uncontrollable. Taunts can come from almost anyone at almost any time. You never know when the student sitting next to you in the lunch room is going to pull out a Snickers bar. Significant events, such as death, separation, divorce, or even a new sibling, can also be stressors.

Researchers differentiate between two kinds of stressors—daily hassles and major life events. Here are some examples:

EXAMPLES OF DAILY HASSLES	EXAMPLES OF MAJOR LIFE EVENTS
Getting teased	Changing jobs
Failing to find flattering clothes to wear	Moving
Misplacing keys	Conflict in a major relationship
Being late	Serious illness or injury
Performing poorly at a task or a sport	Death of a loved one
Failing to understand something	
Worrying about someone else's problems	
Weather problems	
Traffic problems	
Being criticized (recall the stereotype of overweight kids)	
Forgetting something	

It's possible that you and your child experienced some discomfort from reading this list as you recalled reactions to events like these. Talk about these with your child. Discuss whether it might affect your child's food choices if she were teased, interrupted from completing something, or grappling with a major life event. Would her activity routine still go according to plan?

Creating

the

Sierras

Solution

Environment

in

Your

Home

—

72

Help Your Child Develop Resilience

Psychologists who have studied stress management for decades know a great deal about those who prosper when faced with stressors. The Lauren E.'s of the world, like the athletes who perform well under pressure, are described as "resilient" or "hardy."

Resilient (or hardy) people not only avoid harm from stressors, they often flourish under this pressure. Dr. Suzanne Kobasa's research indicates that hardy people exhibit the "three Cs": commitment, control, and challenge. Those who are committed to their lives and work, who believe they can control their fate, and who see stressors as positive challenges end up managing stress quite effectively.

Exhibiting commitment means giving it your all, not just phoning it in. Many LTWCs exhibit remarkable levels of commitment. Henry E. is a good example.

> I would say I was a model kid at AOS. I worked as hard as I could whenever I was exercising. I was thinking to myself, "Well, if I'm here, I'm gonna do it. I'm gonna work as hard as I can," and that turned into, "I can do this, and I'm doing this for me."
>
> —HENRY E., SIXTEEN, COLUMBUS, OHIO
> INITIAL WEIGHT LOSS: 108 POUNDS IN SIX MONTHS
> SUSTAINED WEIGHT LOSS: 108 POUNDS FOR OVER 1½ YEARS

Exhibiting control means taking ownership of the problem, as you've obviously done by buying this book to help your overweight child. Lauren S.'s mom is a good example. She refused to accept that her child was destined to remain overweight.

> I had always tried to get her to eat healthier, had worked with her, had gone to Weight Watchers with her, had gone to nutritionists with her, had exercised with her; we ran the gamut, up and down.
>
> —TERI S., MOTHER OF LAUREN S., FIFTEEN, CALABASAS, CALIFORNIA
> LAUREN'S INITIAL WEIGHT LOSS: FIFTY POUNDS IN FOUR MONTHS
> LAUREN'S TOTAL WEIGHT LOSS: SIXTY-FOUR POUNDS FOR MORE THAN ONE YEAR

> *I don't always catch myself and that's probably why I've gained back a few pounds. But I know it's a lifelong thing. As long as I keep at it and persevere and do my program, I know it'll be all right.*
>
> —DAN B., SEVENTEEN, MESA, ARIZONA
>   INITIAL WEIGHT LOSS: 146 POUNDS IN TEN MONTHS
>   SUSTAINED WEIGHT LOSS: 133 POUNDS FOR OVER 1½ YEARS

Exhibiting challenge means you keep looking for solutions until you find them. You don't give in to hopelessness, and refuse to give up despite previous failures.

Ask questions that develop resilience. To help your young weight controller adopt this approach, teach him to ask himself questions that put him in charge of his stressors. Talk in terms of challenges and opportunities rather than promoting complaints and problems in whiny and hopeless tones. Add these questions to your family's daily conversations at home.

- What can I do to eliminate this stressor?
- How can I look at this problem as an opportunity for change and growth?
- In what ways does this stressor teach me something about my life?
- How can I use this situation to improve my functioning or competence?

Teach Your Child to Solicit Support from Friends and Family

Decades of research show that those with strong relationships suffer fewer medical and emotional problems than those who are more isolated. Simply put, we do better at almost anything when we're surrounded by people who actively show they care. Because the support of friends and family can play such an important role in stress management, one great stress-management skill is knowing when and whom to ask for help. Encourage your child to learn and ask for the different ways that others can show them support.

Teach him to ask for emotional support. Listen and talk things over to let

Creating
the
Sierras
Solution
Environment
in
Your
Home

74

your child know you understand. Allow your child to talk freely about problems and private thoughts. Show confidence and provide encouragement. Positive, nonjudgmental experiences like these will encourage him to continue to seek out emotional support from other good listeners in addition to you.

Coach her to ask for informational support. Give advice your child can count on. Provide resources that are useful. Help your child solve problems by suggesting various solutions from which she can choose. Let her have control of the information and encourage her to seek out support from other available resources—experienced weight controllers, research librarians, food labels, reliable websites, and so on.

Help him understand the material support you provide. You undoubtedly already provide food, shelter, clothing, and education for your child. Continue to be generous, but help him to recognize that these are all ways you show your love and support for him. Help him develop a greater appreciation for the other resources for this kind of support—his teachers, grandparents, friends, and relatives.

Keep the support coming. Once you've become more tuned in to signs of stress from your weight controller, and have responded by providing more support, your child may start asking you to spend more time with her. If you ever feel annoyed about having to manage these requests for extra attention, try thinking about it as if you're depositing money in a savings account. Providing a bit of extra support for your child now will likely pay off down the road.

Use Stress Inoculation

University of Waterloo psychologist Dr. Don Meichenbaum has developed a useful approach for handling major stressors. Called "stress inoculation," this two-phase technique builds "psychological antibodies" of stress resistance by helping your child separate problematic emotions, like anger and anxiety, from stressors.

First, learn about the stressor. In this phase of stress inoculation, fear of the unknown is tackled head-on by gathering information about the stressor. For example, a child approaching her first day of high school might be

Sierras Solution Success Story—Lawrence M.

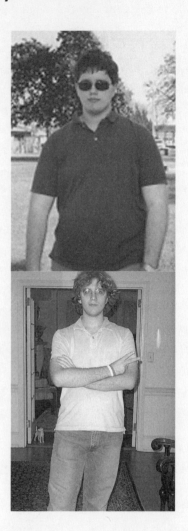

Lawrence grew up with three siblings in an affluent home in Manhattan, the son of two prominent lawyers. Diagnosed with multiple allergies at a young age, he remembers his mom keeping a vigilant eye on his eating. Lawrence often felt angry and out of control, and his grades declined as his weight increased.

Because of my allergies, I was not allowed to eat many of the same things my friends were. I found opportunities to sneak foods, and it became a comfort to know that my parents didn't have complete control.

My grades were constantly in jeopardy. My allergies would kick in all the time and cause me to do even worse academically. I almost never invited my friends over—I preferred reading or watching TV. I was gaining weight at the time we would sometimes play games with Shirts versus Skins, so my dislike for sports intensified into hatred and shame. I would come home at 6:00 p.m. from sports every night and collapse from the fatigue, exertion, and the emotional drain of arguing with my school, teachers, and parents.

I changed schools in ninth grade to a far more flexible environment (no coat-and-tie dress code, coed, and optional sports). For a year, I excelled and was happy. I weighed nearly 220 pounds, but I made good friends, got into interesting classes, and got to hang out with girls. Unfortunately, at the end of that year, the only girl that I had truly liked left after politely rejecting me for being a cynical jerk. That hurt.

(continued)

The next year, all of my grades declined. I went on Weight Watchers, tried exercising with my mom (I *hated* that) and even went to France for a semester to see if that helped. I reached my all-time-high weight—286 pounds.

After going through the AOS program, a lot has changed. My parents don't argue and yell at me anymore; my dad and I talked about our lack of time together and are prepared to change it; my classmates were all amazed by my weight loss; and I no longer see everyone and everything through a pessimistic haze. I feel stronger. I've prioritized and organized my life a bit and I've tested some of my opinions about myself. I was delighted to find that they were wrong.

I actually have a life now. I make an impact on my school. I have even been flirted with by some girls at parties and such. I didn't get together with any of them and I didn't quite catch the third one's name, but still—it's progress.

—LAWRENCE M., FIFTEEN, NEW YORK, NEW YORK
    INITIAL WEIGHT LOSS: NINETY POUNDS IN SEVEN MONTHS
    SUSTAINED WEIGHT LOSS: EIGHTY-SIX POUNDS FOR OVER FOUR MONTHS

terrified. She might have no idea what happens between classes or how she'll get from one end of school to the other. You could help her by getting a map of the classrooms, charting her course between classes, and doing a dry run (with the help of the school staff). Alternately, perhaps your daughter could ask a kindhearted older teen to answer her questions and be a mentor to her in the early months of school.

Then use coping self-statements. We all talk to ourselves, at least sometimes. You may have done so when you took your first dive off of a diving board or made your first public speech. Perhaps you made self-statements like "C'mon, you can do it," or "Go for it." Research shows that such self-statements are actually quite helpful when facing challenges of all kinds. Vicki M. uses this skill.

I'll be sitting and I'll be wanting to eat something 'cause I'll be really stressed out. But I'll just walk away and I'll just think, "You don't need it. It's not worth it." It's just a mental thing. I have to tell myself that I don't need it.

—VICKI M., FOURTEEN, FAIRFAX, VIRGINIA
INITIAL WEIGHT LOSS: SIXTY-SIX POUNDS IN SIX MONTHS
SUSTAINED WEIGHT LOSS: FIFTY-FOUR POUNDS FOR SIX ADDITIONAL
MONTHS

In the second part of stress inoculation, people facing such challenges use four types of self-statements: preparing for the stressor, confronting and handling the stressor, coping with feelings at critical moments, and rewarding oneself for successful coping. Here are some examples of these four types of self-statements that can be used to manage almost any stressor.

SELF-STATEMENTS WHEN PREPARING FOR A STRESSOR

- What do I have to do?
- I can create a plan to deal with this.
- Thinking about what I have to do is certainly better than getting nervous about it.
- Worrying won't help. Planning will.
- My anxiety tells me that I have a challenge facing me.
- I can learn from this.
- Remain logical and calm.

SELF-STATEMENTS WHEN CONFRONTING AND HANDLING THE STRESSOR

- I can handle this.
- I can meet this challenge.
- Just take it one step at a time; follow the plan.
- Beat the fear. Think of what I am doing.
- Relax. I'm in control. Just take a slow, deep breath.
- My tension just tells me to follow my plan, deal with this challenge.
- I can eat safe foods as part of my plan.

Creating
the
Sierras
Solution
Environment
in
Your
Home

———

78

Self-Statements When Coping with Feelings at Critical Moments

- When tension comes, just pause and breathe slowly.
- Focus on the present. Now, what do I have to do?
- I've handled this before and I can manage it now.
- I'll rate my fear from one to ten and then watch it change.
- I'll just keep the tension manageable; I won't worry about eliminating it altogether.
- I can do this. It will be over in a certain amount of time.
- Okay, keep focused on what I want to do.
- This is not the worst thing that can happen.
- Remember, I don't have to handle this perfectly, just reasonably well.
- Focus on sensations: coldness, warmth, smells, touch, taste, sights, and sounds.
- Think about other times and places. Good feelings come with good thoughts.
- I'm in control.
- If I'm going to overeat, I'll eat more of the low-fat stuff; I won't eat high-fat food.

Self-Statements When Rewarding Yourself for Successful Coping

- Nice going! I was able to do it.
- It wasn't as tough as I expected.
- Wait till I tell [a friend, a family member] about it.
- I'm making progress.
- My plan worked.
- I'm learning all the time.
- It's my thinking that creates anxiety. When I control my self-statements, I can control my anxiety.
- I'm doing better each time I use these self-statements.
- I'm really pleased with my progress.

By using these self-statements, your child can begin to actively cope with stressors and become more hardy and resilient. To practice this technique, ask your weight controller to pick a stressor and work through these self-statements with you.

Try Cued Relaxation

Everyday life holds many opportunities to strengthen your child's stress-response skills. Increasing relaxation can help decrease negative reactions to stressors, such as daily hassles. Decreased stress can mean fewer triggers for emotional eating. In cued relaxation, a person reminds himself to release his tension every time he experiences a cue, such as a ringing cell phone, drinking water, reaching for a wallet, brushing hair, or applying makeup. When the cue occurs, the person takes a few seconds to use a relaxation technique. Consider these examples.

CUE: RINGING CELL PHONE

1. Cell phone rings.
2. Answer phone.
3. Start breathing slowly and rhythmically.
4. During the call, focus on continuing to breathe in a relaxed manner.
5. After the call, take another few seconds to breathe deeply, slowly, and rhythmically.

CUE: DRINKING WATER OR DIET SODA

1. Begin drinking.
2. Focus on the fluid and the sounds and sights of it.
   - What color is it?
   - What, specifically, does it sound like as you drink?
   - Concentrate on the texture of the fluid as it enters your mouth and goes down your throat.
3. Create a vivid image that involves water. For example:
   - You are on a beach in the summertime and you are watching a lake gently flow to the shore and retreat from the shore.
   - You are hiking on a mountain and you come upon a beautiful

Creating
the
Sierras
Solution
Environment
in
Your
Home
—
80

waterfall. You are watching the water flow and beat down on the rocks below. You are listening to the sounds and smelling the air.

4. Take a few minutes to stay in the image, keeping it vivid, using all of your senses to enliven the imagery.

CUE: REACHING FOR YOUR WALLET

1. After your hand makes contact with the wallet, remind yourself to relax.
2. Tense and then relax some of the muscles in your hand and arm. Tense and relax those muscles at least twice.
3. Pay attention to the change in sensation from the tense to the relaxed state for each muscle group that you use. Focus on the relaxed state for a few seconds and try to bring that sense of relaxation from the top of your head through your eyes and down to the rest of your body.

Including these moments of relaxation during the day will help your child tune in to his own intuitive stress-management ability, as well as hone these skills so he can tap them during times of heightened stress.

You're Ready to Start

This is the moment you've been preparing for. You've learned about your child's unique biology and how it presents the greatest roadblock to weight loss. You have a sense of how "everything else"—the environment, family dynamics, and personal habits—can, in fact, be managed in the face of these biological roadblocks. You've already begun to create an environment in your home that will support your child's success on the Sierras Solution program. Armed with the full understanding of both the scope and the potential rewards of your mutual challenge, you and your weight controller are now ready to start implementing the three Simple Changes of the Sierras Solution.

Help Your Child
Manage Stress:
Tips and Strategies
for Overcoming
Emotional Eating
———

PART 3

The Sierras
Solution Program

Chapter 6

The Three Simple Changes:
An Overview of the
Sierras Solution Program

I was amazed that the Sierras Solution seemed so easy and flexible. It's something I can really live with and I have been living with it for many months now outside of AOS.

—COURTNEY D., SEVENTEEN, NORWICH, VERMONT
   INITIAL WEIGHT LOSS: FIFTY-FOUR POUNDS IN FIVE MONTHS
   SUSTAINED WEIGHT LOSS: FORTY-EIGHT POUNDS FOR OVER FOUR
   MONTHS

The Sierras Solution relies on three guiding principles.

First, all elements of the Sierras Solution have a solid foundation in *science*. We rely on peer-reviewed journal articles as understood by our scientific advisory board and those of us with a substantial background in science.

Second, as far as possible, we keep the primary instructions of the plan *simple*. Simplicity means that these behavioral directives have very clear goals and are easily measured. Keeping track allows weight controllers to determine whether they're accomplishing their goals every day.

Finally, we also use principles and techniques that have a proven long-term track record. In other words, these techniques and ways of thinking are *sustainable*.

The Sierras Solution Is Scientific

Imagine that you or your weight-controller child picked up many of the bestselling diet books from the past few years. If you decided to review all of them and distill their most important and significant bits of advice, you would find a listing that looks something like this:

- Forget about calories; fat is where it's at.
- Forget about fat; protein is where it's at.
- Forget about fat and protein; carbs are where it's at.

Notice any contradictions? If you followed one diet for a while and then tried another, you'd find yourself focusing on opposite things—low carbs on one, then low fat on the other. If you tried following all of these rules at the same time, you'd be left drinking water and that's about it. That shows the confusing nature of these nonscientifically based approaches.

These quick fixes and quirky meal plans just don't work. It's true that most people who attempt one or more of these regimens over a short period of time will experience some weight loss. But people can't sustain such quirky combinations of foods for long periods of time. It takes too much effort to do this, and such unusual programs fail to fit into life's various activities (parties, vacations, restaurants).

The Sierras Solution was developed with the help of a distinguished scientific advisory board and distilled from hundreds of studies published in *Obesity, Journal of the American Medical Association, New England Journal of Medicine, Behavior Therapy*, and many other authoritative peer-reviewed scientific journals. These journals provide a wealth of information about weight loss and related factors, the vast majority of which is generally unknown to the public.

Dedicated to formulating and fine-tuning an approach that works in the real world, we've taken this wealth of information and field-tested our approach by administering similar programs to thousands of young people in our clinics, camps, and schools. The Sierras Solution program represents both the best current scientific knowledge and our collective clinical experience about how to lose weight and keep it off, enjoyably and comfortably.

The Sierras Solution Is Simple

Most weight controllers have tried to lose weight by following various complicated diets. But decades of research have shown that complex diets are hard to remember and hard to follow, especially over an extended period of time. The more complex the rules are, the more excuses you have not to follow them. Someone could fill a book with all the crazy food decisions people on diets have made by rationalizing their way through complex diet rules.

In contrast, the Simple Changes—the three simple, yet profound, goals—of the Sierras Solution are:

- Eat as little fat as possible, with a goal of fewer than 20 grams of fat a day.
- Stay as active as possible and wear a pedometer, with the goal of at least ten thousand steps per day.
- Self-monitor: keep a record of your eating and exercise every day, or at least 75 percent of the time.

The simplicity of these ideas strikes most overweight kids and adults as extraordinary. Most serial dieters are used to numerous restrictions about what they can eat, what time of day they can eat, and a variety of often absurdly Byzantine directives.

In essence, the Simple Changes of the Sierras Solution are ideal goals because all three are action oriented, measurable, and associated with immediate feedback.

Each Simple Change is action-oriented. The first change directs weight controllers to eat very little fat; the second change directs weight con-

> *That's one of the things I love about the Sierras Solution. There's nothing confusing about it. When I was five years old, I could have understood it!*
>
> —Jarrett F., twelve,
>   St. Charles, Illinois
> Initial weight loss:
> eighty-nine pounds in nine months
> Sustained weight loss:
> eighty pounds for over 1½ years

trollers to stay active and wear a pedometer; the third change directs weight controllers to create a daily record about their eating and exercise.

Each Simple Change provides very clear, easily measured end points. Tallying up daily grams of fat is something that anyone can do. A pedometer counts up your steps and reports your results at the end of the day. And if all food is monitored for the day, then it's counted as a good self-monitoring day.

Each Simple Change has feedback built in. LTWCs look up fat grams as they eat throughout a day. They review the number on their pedometer after taking a walk or to check on their progress. They look at their self-monitoring records as they enter new information throughout each day. This process of tracking helps connect these critical actions to both short-term and longer-term goals. As your teenager eats lunch, he will write down the content of the lunch and record fat grams in a self-monitoring journal. This process reminds him of his short-term daily goals (fewer than 20 fat grams, and consistent self-monitoring). These short-term goals are directly linked to the longer-term goal of weight loss.

The Sierras Solution Is Sustainable

Diets don't work in the long run. They're too complicated and they restrict freedom too much. Temporary success is likely, but long-term success is very unlikely.

Sustainability requires a number of elements. Simple rules are easier to follow, and therefore more sustainable. Approaches that provide more freedom and choice are more sustainable. But dieters know that they face another major issue in sustaining a diet over months and years—the inevitable "violation."

Diets tend to fall apart after dieters have particularly challenging days and really deviate from their plans. Because they realize they've "violated" the principles of their plans, many dieters will give up the plan completely, in order to avoid feeling bad about themselves.

What if you were following a diet that forbade eating carbohydrates and you quickly ate a taboo food like a bagel? You could either feel bad about this violation, or you could decide that you were taking a break from the diet—perhaps even a permanent break. If you're taking a break, you don't have to feel bad about eating that forbidden food—and, lo and behold, you've given up on your efforts to change.

The Sierras Solution avoids generating this reaction by focusing on goals for each day. The key daily goals are to eat as little fat as possible (fewer than 20 grams maximum), attain ten thousand steps or more, and self-monitor consistently. If some of these goals aren't achieved on Monday, the Sierras Solution teaches weight controllers to start over with the same goals when the sun rises on Tuesday. This approach is more effective at sustaining efforts over time.

Sustainability is also greatly enhanced by developing what we call a "healthy obsession." This healthy obsession is how we define the thorough and sustained commitment to lifestyle change that is required to beat the biological and environmental forces opposing weight control. Admittedly, and to positive ends, this healthy obsession creates a bit of discomfort when the three Simple Changes are not achieved in a given day. However, this unhappiness can be washed away by renewed efforts to change at any point in time. We'll discuss how to nurture and promote this healthy obsession in chapter 10.

Family support is also critical in sustaining the Sierras Solution. We know from our own research that weight controllers do better when families follow the Sierras Solution at home. Put differently, it's the rare fifteen-year-old who can successfully maintain her weight if the family is ordering pizza every other night, and high-fat fast food twice a week. Please follow the Sierras Solution as much as possible. This kind of modeling provides

I keep close track of my weight and I make sure I take action when it gets too high. The number 210 is a very scary number for me, for example. When I hit that number or get close to it, I take action. I start exercising every day and eating incredibly well every single day until I drive it back down.

—HENRY E., SIXTEEN,
COLUMBUS, OHIO
INITIAL WEIGHT LOSS:
108 POUNDS IN SIX MONTHS
SUSTAINED WEIGHT LOSS:
108 POUNDS FOR OVER 1½ YEARS

incredibly powerful support. We will review in detail how to do this in chapter 7.

To give your child the opportunity to experience the best results, we ask you and other family members to begin making the three Simple Changes along with your weight controller. And remember, all three Simple Changes are likely to be beneficial for the health of all family members, including those who have never had a weight problem.

Let's talk about how you can start right now.

Getting Started with Three Simple Changes

First off, make sure you have your notebook nearby. You've already captured your feelings, goals, and commitments for the program. You'll probably want to refer back to your Decision Balance Sheet and all of the other thoughts you've captured in your notebook during the first few weeks.

Then, we recommend that you also make at least eighty-four photocopies of the Self-Monitoring Journal in appendix 5—that's enough for one SMJ a day for you and your weight controller for the first six weeks of the plan. (Add forty-two extra copies for each additional family member.) But if you'd like to use your notebook—or even a PDA or computer—instead, that's fine, too.

Finally, decide how you'll approach the plan. You have many different options. That's the beauty of the plan—it's so flexible because it's so simple.

Do you want all the information first, before you start? Some weight controllers and their parents prefer to get a handle on the entire program before they start. If that sounds like you, read through the next three chapters with your weight controller. Once you have a handle on the whole program, you can move to the next step.

Are you eager to get going? If you're eager to get going, turn to the Week 1 shopping list on page 301, grab your keys, and take your weight controller to the grocery store to stock up. Stop by the sporting-goods store to pick up a pedometer. Check out the menu plan for Week 1 (see chapter 11, page 209), plan some time to fit in your ten thousand steps tomorrow, and get ready to start with breakfast in the morning.

Once you're under way, you can turn back to the book and read chapters

7, 8, and 9 to better understand the rationale for, and the practice of, each individual Simple Change while you're following the meal plan.

Aren't much for meal plans? If you don't like to follow a prescribed plan and you prefer to design your own meals, feel free to do so—just make sure they are based on the nutritional principles of the program set out in chapter 7 and the substitution lists on page 121.

Want to take it slow and steady? If you prefer to ease into the program, no problem. You might want to add one Simple Change per week. We suggest that, in this case, you start with Simple Change 3, self-monitoring, first. When you begin on the Sierras Solution, it's very difficult to track your fat grams unless you're marking it down in some way. (Of course, you'll soon become a pro!) In Week 2, you can move on to Simple Change 1, limiting your fat intake to fewer than 20 grams a day, and in Week 3, add in Simple Change 2, achieving your daily goal of ten thousand steps.

By the first day of Week 4, you'll have the entire plan under your belt, and you'll begin to see how these Simple Changes can make a tremendous difference in your weight controller's life—and yours, too. At our Academy of the Sierras and Wellspring programs, it's not uncommon for new weight controllers to lose more than four pounds per week during the first few weeks on the plan. However, keep in mind that the most successful outpatient programs achieve an average of one-half to one pound of weight loss per week. Losing one pound per week is achievable once the entire plan is working for you.

In the next three chapters, you'll learn all about the three Simple Changes of the Sierras Solution. Along the way, you'll discover how you can establish a foundation for lifelong weight control for yourself and your entire family.

Chapter 7

Simple Change #1
Eat Fewer Than 20 Grams of
Fat Every Day

Low-fat eating has gotten a bad rap.

Ever since the advent of the low-carb craze, low-fat eating was shoved to the side, scoffed at, even blamed for the upward trend in obesity.

Well, we think that's ludicrous, and here's why: dozens of studies over the past half century have clearly suggested the superiority of a very low-fat approach to weight loss. We believe it's high time for very low-fat eating to come out of the shadows and claim its rightful spot as the clear winner in the weight-loss wars.

In Simple Change #1, the Sierras Solution takes all of the available science and boils it down to one easily understandable, easy-to-implement weight-loss strategy: Eat as little fat as you can, with a daily maximum of 20 grams.

Before you start lamenting the loss of fat in your life, please know that the Sierras Solution eating plan is nothing like the bland low-fat cooking of yore. Just a few days of eating the recipes and following the menu plans found in chapters 11 and 12 will convince both you and your weight controller that you'll barely miss the fat. In fact, like most of our LTWCs, after a while you may even start to feel grossed out by fatty foods!

The truth is that successful weight controllers do not have to give up much of anything to enjoy a full range of wonderful taste sensations. When you adopt Simple Change #1, you learn that there are literally *thousands* of foods and methods of preparation that will allow you to eat delicious, satisfying, healthful foods that also help you lose weight. Let's take a look at the convincing science behind Simple Change 1 and why the debate over "what really works" is finally over.

The Science of Low-Fat Eating

The verdict is in. Dozens of scientific studies have shown that high-fat foods lead to weight gain. Low-fat diets work. (And low-carb diets do *not*—contrary to what you may have heard.)

Consider some of the most important scientific findings.

More fat equals more calories. Fats are more than twice as calorie-dense as carbohydrates and proteins. The more fat you eat, the higher your caloric intake. It's as simple as that.

The more fat you eat, the fewer calories your body burns. Dietary fats are also stored as additional body fat more easily than carbs or protein are. To turn one hundred calories of very high-fat foods like butter or bacon into body fat, your body expends only about three calories of energy. That means that ninety-seven of the one hundred calories end up in your fat cells. But in order to turn one hundred calories of spaghetti into fat, the body has to expend about twenty-three calories. Turning carbohydrates into fat is much more complicated, since the body has to change the carbohydrate into a number of other chemical compounds in order to process it. By contrast, it takes very little energy for the body to transform foods that already start out as fat into body fat.

Fat is more fattening for overweight and formerly overweight people. When overweight or formerly overweight people eat food with fat in it, fat is transported more directly into storage in the fat cells. When never-overweight people eat fat, more fat goes into muscles to be used more immediately for energy. These processes have been demonstrated in animals, and researchers believe the same pattern applies to humans.

The hormones of overweight and formerly overweight people react more to fat. Overweight and formerly overweight people also have a greater sensitivity to fat than their never-overweight peers. This means a higher level

> *The scientific verdict is in. If your child is going to become a long-term weight controller, he has to say good-bye to fat.*

of reactivity at the cellular level. Specifically, overweight people salivate more and secrete more insulin in the presence of appealing high-fat foods. High-fat diets also may make you produce problematic levels of hormones like leptin and ghrelin, and reduce the amount of insulin transmitted to the brain. All of these hormonal effects can make you hungrier and more likely to eat more and gain weight.

High-fat foods are more fattening than high-carb foods—even with the same calories. Studies with small animals show that diets that are high in fat can make you gain weight. A high-fat diet will make you gain more weight than a high-carb diet—even when the diets have the same number of calories. If you feed some groups of rats one thousand calories of high-fat rat chow, they will gain more weight than rats fed one thousand calories of high-carbohydrate (but low-fat) rat chow. Even high-fat "weight-loss diets" prevent rats from losing weight—but their brethren who eat low-fat diets with the same number of calories lose substantial amounts of weight.

Eating some fat makes you eat more food. Researchers have found that eating foods that are high in fat may encourage overeating because they generally increase your hunger and diminish your feelings of fullness (or satiety). Fat foods stimulate an internal reaction that's called the "endogenous opioid system," a powerful internal pleasure system.

The more fat you eat, the more likely you'll gain excess weight. Studies with large numbers of young people and adults show that those who eat higher-fat diets are more likely to become obese over time.

Weight controllers who maintain very low-fat diets keep weight off the longest. Perhaps the most compelling studies come from an ambitious project called the National Weight Control Registry. The registry, started in 1994 by psychologists Dr. James Hill and Dr. Rena Wing, includes more than five thousand people who have verifiably lost at least thirty pounds and kept it off for at least one year. Researchers found that these successful weight controllers eat about 33 percent less fat than average Americans. They also consume about ten times more carbohydrates than the Atkins low-carb diet recommends. Follow-up studies have shown that when these masters of weight control eat a bit more fat and decrease their activities a little, they tend to regain some weight. Meanwhile, eating more carbohydrates did not predict weight regain.

How Much Fat Does Your Family Eat?

Before you and your weight controller say good-bye (and good riddance) to fat, it's helpful to know just how much you've been eating. The following quiz can help you determine your own eating and cooking patterns.

EATING SURVEY

Check the answer that best describes the way you have been eating over the past month.

1. **How many ounces of meat, fish or poultry do you usually eat?***
   __ 1. I do not eat meat, fish, or poultry.
   __ 2. I eat three ounces or less per day.
   __ 3. I eat four to six ounces per day.
   __ 4. I eat seven or more ounces per day.

2. **How much cheese do you eat per week?**
   __ 1. I do not eat cheese.
   __ 2. I eat whole-milk cheese less than once a week and/or I use only low-fat cheese.
   __ 3. I eat whole-milk cheese (such as cheddar, Swiss, or Monterey jack) once or twice per week.
   __ 4. I eat whole-milk cheese three or more times per week.

Simple Change #1:
Eat Fewer Than
20 Grams of
Fat Every Day

* Three ounces of meat, fish, or chicken is any *ONE* of the following: one regular fast-food–type (small) hamburger, one chicken breast, one chicken leg (thigh and drumstick), one pork chop, or three slices of presliced lunch meat.

3. **What type of milk do you use?**

___ 1. I use only skim or 1 percent milk or I don't use milk.

___ 2. I usually use skim milk or 1 percent milk but use others occasionally.

___ 3. I usually use 2 percent or whole milk.

4. **How many visible egg yolks do you use per week?**

___ 1. I avoid all egg yolks or use less than one per week and/or use only egg substitute.

___ 2. I eat one to two egg yolks per week.

___ 3. I eat three or more egg yolks per week.

5. **How often do you consume these meats: regular-fat hamburger, bologna, salami, hot dogs, corned beef, spareribs, sausage, bacon, braunschweiger, or liver? Do not count low-fat cuts of meat.**

___ 1. I do not eat any of those meats.

___ 2. I eat them about once per week or less.

___ 3. I eat them about two to four times per week.

___ 4. I eat more than four servings per week.

6. **How many commercially baked goods, such as cake, cookies, coffee cake, sweet rolls, and doughnuts, and how much regular ice cream do you usually eat? Do not count low-fat versions.**

___ 1. I do not eat commercially baked goods or ice cream.

___ 2. I eat commercially baked goods or ice cream once per week or less.

___ 3. I eat commercially baked goods or ice cream two to four times per week.

___ 4. I eat commercially baked goods or ice cream more than four times per week.

7. **What is the main type of fat you use in cooking?**

___ 1. I use nonstick spray or I do not use fat in cooking.

___ 2. I use liquid oil, such as safflower, sunflower, corn, soybean, and olive oil.

___ 3. I use margarine.

___ 4. I use butter, shortening, bacon drippings, or lard.

8. **How often do you eat snack foods, such as regular-fat chips, fries, or party crackers? Do not count fat-free or low-fat versions.**

___ 1. I do not eat those snack foods.

___ 2. I eat one serving or less of those snacks per week.

___ 3. I eat those snacks two to four times per week.

___ 4. I eat those snack foods more than four times per week.

9. **What spread do you usually use on bread and vegetables?**

___ 1. I do not use any spread.

___ 2. I use diet or light margarine.

___ 3. I use margarine.

___ 4. I use butter.

10. **How often do you eat candy bars, chocolate, or nuts as a snack?**

___ 1. Less than once per week.

___ 2. One to three times per week.

___ 3. More than three times per week.

11. **When you use recipes or convenience foods, how often are they low fat?**

___ 1. Almost always.

___ 2. Usually.

___ 3. Sometimes.

___ 4. Seldom or never.

12. **When you eat away from home, how often do you choose low-fat foods?**

___ 1. Almost always.

___ 2. Usually

___ 3. Sometimes.

___ 4. Seldom or never.

Note: This questionnaire was developed by B. M. Retzlaff, A. A. Dowdy, C. E. Walden, V. E. Bovbjerg, and R. H. Knopp of the Northwest Lipid Research Clinic at the University of Washington, Seattle. It was first published by them in the 1997 *American Journal of Public Health* (volume 87, 181–85) and is reprinted here with permission of the American Public Health Association.

Simple Change #1:
Eat Fewer Than
20 Grams of
Fat Every Day

——

Add the numbers of your responses together to form a total. For example, if you choose the option "I eat three ounces of meat, fish, or poultry," for question 1, your score for that item would be a 2. The highest score you can get on this survey is 45 and the lowest is 12.

According to the researchers who developed this questionnaire, a score of 24 corresponds to a relatively high-fat, high-cholesterol diet. The average score for a group of 310 adult Americans surveyed in the initial research was 30, equal to about 82 grams of fat per day. How did you score compared to the average score of 30?

AOS students rate their diets prior to coming to AOS as quite high in fat, averaging a score of 33 on the quiz, which probably translates to an average intake of about 110 fat grams per day—significantly higher than the national average of 82 fat grams per day.

Before they enroll at AOS, students often eat high-fat meats, cheeses, bakery items, and dairy products. Consider how much fat twelve-year-old Jarrett, who has sustained his eighty-pound weight loss for over a year, used to eat before AOS.

> *Breakfast, I'd get two packages of Pop Tarts and some chocolate milk. Or I'd get two bowls of cereal filled to the brim, sugary cereal with whole milk. For lunch it'd be the cafeteria food. If I was still hungry, kids knew who to give their extra food to. After school I'd snack on leftovers or chips. For dinner, Dad and I got pizza or we went to a burger place or sports bar. Almost every night, we'd get ice cream.*

We hear stories like this every day. Remember, many young people can eat just like this and never develop a weight problem. But for those who are biologically predisposed to gain weight, eating high-fat foods regularly creates a lot of excess weight, particularly in those who aren't very active. And anyone who eats like this risks developing a range of health problems over time.

The good news is that these patterns can change. Following the Sierras Solution program will teach you and your weight controller how to reduce your fat intake dramatically and permanently. For over a year since leaving AOS, the alumni profiled in this book have continued to eat about the same amount of fat that they consumed while at AOS. Their success delights us because it points to a strong family commitment. LTWCs not only change their own eating patterns but those of their families, too.

Go as Low Fat as You Can

Your new mantra for fat is "Go as low as you can go." You and your weight controller will improve your ability to control your weight by striving for a goal of no fat (zero fat grams) while knowing that you're okay if you stick with 20 fat grams or less per day.

Don't worry that you won't be getting enough fat. Even apples and carrots have small amounts of fat. Bread has fat. It's impossible to get to zero fat, and dietitians recommend a minimum of 3 to 5 grams of fat per day for health. But shooting for no fat and settling for less than 20 grams per day works well. (For infants and toddlers less than two years old, this doesn't work. Check with your pediatrician for recommendations.)

How do you do this? Simple, really. You hunt down all kinds of fat and eliminate it. Grams of fat per serving are right on the packages of most foods. While counting calories involves large, cumbersome numbers, everyone can aim for zero and count to twenty!

One reference that we find indispensable is a simple nutrition counter book. The bookstores are full of them, and any one will probably work. For the Sierras Solution, we recommend the pocket-sized book *Calorie King,* a colorful and user-friendly guide that lists the fat and calories in every food you can imagine, including menu items from most restaurant chains. Purchasing and relying on a nutrition counter book is a huge help in making the first Simple Change simple and sustainable.

Using this kind of a reference tool, your weight controller will become an expert in just a few weeks. All you have to do is add up the fat grams in everything you eat, aim for zero, and work hard to stay under 20. That's it.

What About "Good" and "Bad" Fats?

Great question. It's true that certain types of "bad" fat—such as saturated fats and trans fats found in fried and many processed foods—create more cardiovascular health problems than other types of "good" fat—such as polyunsaturated fats found in olive oil and peanut oil. So, if you had a choice, you'd want to eat the good fats instead of the bad fats. However, two points are worth noting with regard to weight control. First, successful weight controllers generally eat so little fat that the type of fat becomes rather important. The studies that show the dangers of eating bad fat are based on

Simple Change #1:
Eat Fewer Than
20 Grams of
Fat Every Day

—

99

Sierras Solution Success Story

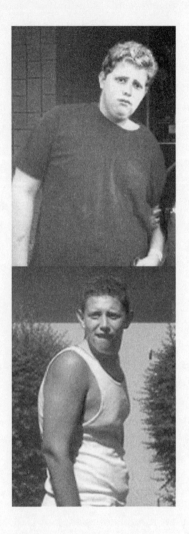

Henry's mother recalls that his first word was "more." He developed a weight problem as a child and tried numerous diets, but kept gaining the weight back. Before coming to AOS, Henry felt so defeated that he thought it would be best to keep eating a lot so that he could qualify for bariatric surgery. Now his motto is "I can do anything I want with my life."

I had been heavy my entire life. In high school, I thought everyone made fun of me behind my back, but it was really my mind, overthinking things. I used tennis to cope with my unhappiness and I didn't gain weight because of the tremendous amount of time I put into the game. I had a tennis coach who became like a second mother to me. When she left spontaneously, without warning, I was devastated that she didn't say good-bye. I gave up on my tennis, something I loved more than anything at the time. That's when I began to binge eat—I would eat over fifteen thousand calories a day and over a thousand grams of fat a day. Five months later, I'd gained over sixty pounds and I weighed over three hundred pounds.

I was in complete denial. At a certain point when I was gaining the weight, I thought, "Well, if I just keep eating, I'll be big enough to get the surgery." When my parents told me about AOS, I said, "I'm not one of them. I don't need to be." Then when I got there I just started working really hard and found that I could eat pretty well and I liked to exercise a lot.

If I hadn't done the program, my future would have been very grim. I

(continued)

would, at this point, probably weigh over four hundred pounds, because of the mind-boggling rate at which I had been gaining weight. Basically, I would be on the fast track to a short and miserable life that would be threatened at an early age due to health reasons.

This program helped me lose over one hundred pounds and my negative self-view. What people think is of no importance to me; what really matters is how I view myself. I no longer feel like people talk about me behind my back and, if they do, I no longer fear what they are saying.

I've now been doing it for so long, I know how to lose weight, and I'm happy with my weight. I am confident in my ability to live a healthy life, to be a long-term weight controller. I also am confident that when I start my senior year at a new school, I will not only be myself in front of other people but I will be proud of who I am.

—HENRY E., SIXTEEN, COLUMBUS, OHIO
INITIAL WEIGHT LOSS: 108 POUNDS IN SIX MONTHS
SUSTAINED WEIGHT LOSS: 108 POUNDS FOR OVER 1½ YEARS

research with people who average many times more fat grams per day compared to successful weight controllers. If someone eats 80 or 100 grams of unhealthy fat per day, then they can expect to develop health problems like heart disease. If someone eats just a few grams of such fat per day, they're probably at low risk for developing such problems. Second, if your child is able to become a successful weight controller, the likelihood of cardiovascular issues down the road diminishes radically. So don't worry very much about whether or not your child eats fats from fish or olive oil versus saturated animal fat from lean chicken or buffalo meat. Your child's health will be vastly improved by losing weight, first and foremost. That weight loss will come from tremendous improvements in the diet (such as much lower consumption of *all* fats, including bad fats) and greatly increased activity levels. Even if your child doesn't lose an ounce, increasing activity consistently greatly reduces the risk of heart disease, cancer, and other killers.

Some people also worry about the source of fats, not just the type of fats. Cornell University professor Colin Campbell emphasized in his remarkable

Simple Change #1:
Eat Fewer Than
20 Grams of
Fat Every Day

—

book *The China Study* that plant-based fats appear to be much better for your long-term health than fats that come from animals. By making Simple Change #1, you and your weight controller will naturally eat more plant-based meals and much less animal fat. So, it's likely your entire family will eat proportionately more "good" fat than ever before.

We believe the highest healthy priority for any overweight child is to become an LTWC. And the research is clear that from a purely weight-control perspective, *a fat is a fat is a fat.*

One tablespoon of peanut oil, lard, corn oil, coconut oil, or butter equals 120 calories and 13.6 fat grams.

All fats contain approximately the same number of calories, and all fats are readily stored by your body as fat. Your understanding of this indisputable fact will simplify the process for your weight controller.

The Optimal Nutrition of a Very Low-Fat Diet

You want to support your weight controller's efforts to lose weight, and you also want to make sure she is getting good nutrition. We do, too! That's why Simple Change #1 is so powerful. The stipulation that weight controllers focus initially on only one aspect of their diet—fat grams—automatically causes them to eat more nutritious foods.

As you'll learn in chapter 11, a typical day of the Sierras Solution eating plan includes three meals and two snacks a day that add up to 1,200 calories, 10 grams of fat, 50 grams of protein, and 30 grams of fiber. You and your weight controller will likely add to that with what we call "uncontrolled" foods, fat-free foods that you can eat to feel comfortable. If you or your weight controller is hungry, you both can have as much uncontrolled food as it takes to help you feel satisfied. See the Uncontrolled Foods and Snacks list on page 124).

In order to follow Simple Change #1 and stay on the plan, you needn't count anything at first but fat grams. There is no caloric goal. Now, granted, a teen could try to "outsmart" Simple Change #1 by eating only Lifesavers and soda, which have no fat. We would say that anyone who tries this is probably still in the shock/ambivalence stage and probably could use a bit of extra help with defining his motivation before he can start on the program. (You could either start again with the Decision Balance Sheet in appendix 2 or see "Provide Structure" on page 193 to help your weight controller overcome shock/ambivalence.)

But as long as you and your weight controller are attempting to eat actual *food* (as opposed to consuming straight sugar), you'll naturally do three other critical things that help control hunger and improve weight control: you'll eat lower-calorie-density foods, eat more fiber, and refrain from drinking calories.

INCREASE YOUR LOW-DENSITY FOODS

If you could eat as much as you wanted in order to feel satisfied, in which of the following meals would you wind up consuming more total calories?

OPTION #1	OPTION #2
Grilled chicken	Soup made from grilled chicken, seasoned white rice, and assorted vegetables
Seasoned white rice	
Assorted vegetables	
One glass of ice water	One glass of ice water

Answer: option #1. A variety of studies suggest you would eat about 20 percent more food and calories when presented in the conventional way (option #1) compared to the soup version (option #2). Option #2 is defined as "low calorie-density" because if you weigh the soup, the number of calories per ounce or gram of the combined chicken, rice, veggies, and water would be relatively low. You'd actually ingest a good deal of water in option #2. In contrast, the chicken dish with a glass of water on the side would be a more energy-dense meal—your number of calories per ounce or gram would be higher—because you took in less water during the meal.

For the same number of calories, you can eat a lot more low-density food. In other words, low-density food weighs more (and has more volume) but has the same calories as high-density food. Eating this way also slows down your digestion, so you feel fuller longer. Studies show that when people add more water to their meals—either with soup or other high-fluid-content

Simple Change #1:
Eat Fewer Than
20 Grams of
Fat Every Day

———

foods like salad or other vegetables—they eat considerably fewer calories. Try some of these tips to increase the fluid content and decrease the energy density of your meals.

- Provide fat-free soups at as many meals as possible.
- Start off every dinner with a salad.
- Serve the vegetables first, before the entrée.
- Put two or three varieties of vegetables on the table at mealtime, and keep the entrée dish on the stove.
- Put out fresh-cut carrots or celery and fat-free dressings (such as ranch or blue cheese) as an after-school snack. A bowl of grapes or snap peas works well, too.
- Model healthy restaurant eating by ordering double portions of vegetables.

ADD MORE FIBER

Health writer Ruth Papazian says that fiber is the Rodney Dangerfield of food: it gets no respect. True, if eaten in large quantities very quickly, fiber (sometimes called roughage) can cause gas, bloating, and other unpleasant side effects. But the pluses of fiber far outweigh the minuses: fiber can decrease appetite, improve weight loss, and reduce the risk of heart disease and some cancers. How is that for respectable?

Populations that consume lots of fiber have relatively few overweight people. In Kenya, Uganda, and Malawi, for example, where less than 15 percent of adults are overweight, people eat more than four times the fiber than we do (60 to 80 grams a day, versus our average of 15 grams a day). Could it be mere coincidence that we eat one-quarter the fiber but have four times the percentage—60 percent—of overweight people than these high-fiber countries?

A substance that's found in plants, fiber has no calories and your body can't digest it. Fiber simply fills up space in your stomach until your body can get rid of it. Fiber also keeps your your intestines clean, sweeping out unhealthy food particles that have been left behind.

Adding fiber is another great tactic to reduce the caloric density of what you're eating. Including a lot of high-fiber vegetables in a meal increases the bulk and weight of the food without influencing the number of calories consumed much at all. Consider what happens when you add lettuce, tomatoes, and bean sprouts to a sandwich and you change the bread from white to whole grain. The veggies might add 30 calories and the change in bread would add no additional calories, but these changes would add about 6 grams of fiber. That extra fiber also increases chewing, promoting increased production of saliva and stomach acids. These fluids and the bulk of the food itself will help fill you up faster and make your belly feel fuller longer—which, of course, helps you eat less.

Most Americans only get 15 grams of fiber a day. Health and nutrition experts recommend that we double that, to 30 grams per day. Eating lots of fiber can really help weight controllers fill up with fewer fat grams. So a great way to help your weight controller meet the Simple Change #1 goal of less than 20 grams of fat per day, you might shoot for 30 or more grams of fiber a day. Here are a few ways to hit that target.

- Choose high-fiber breakfast cereals—one cup of raisin bran, Multi-Bran Chex, or cracked wheat has 8 grams of fiber each.
- Use whole-grain breads for sandwiches; two slices gets you 4 grams of fiber.
- Start eating more beans—bean soups or ¼ cup of baked beans or ½ cup of peas, lentils, or corn all have 5 grams of fiber per serving.
- Enjoy 1 medium white potato with skin, 1 cup of brown rice, or ½ cup of whole-grain pasta, each of which has 4 grams of fiber.
- Pile on three or four servings of veggies or salad, which adds 6 grams extra fiber per serving.
- Snack on fresh fruit, which averages 3 grams of fiber per serving.
- Add color: whole "brown" grains, such as whole-wheat pasta, have much more fiber than refined "white" grains, such as semolina pasta; sweet potatoes have 50 percent more fiber than white ones.
- Eat fresh fruit instead of drinking juice: you'll get more fiber and lower calorie density, you'll spend more time chewing, and you'll enjoy more satisfaction and less hunger.

One last thing—interesting studies have shown that even adding fiber supplements can help you lose weight. One study compared the effects of providing a fiber supplement versus a placebo supplement to overweight participants. The participants who got the fiber supplement lost signifi-

Good Fiber Swaps

Check out how a simple substitution can add up to big gains in fiber.

Low Fiber	High Fiber
White bread (1 slice): 75 calories, 1 gram fat, *0.7 gram fiber*	Whole-grain bread (1 slice): 75 calories, 1 gram fat, *2 grams fiber*
White rice (1 cup, cooked): 240 calories, 0.5 gram fat, *1.6 grams fiber*	Brown rice (1 cup cooked): 220 calories, 1.5 grams fat, *3.2 grams fiber*
Orange juice (one 12-ounce glass): 165 calories, 0 gram fat, *0.5 gram fiber*.	Oranges (2 medium): 140 calories, 0 gram fat, *7.6 grams fiber*

cantly more weight and reported significantly less hunger than the placebo group. Other research suggests that fiber supplementation also improves blood sugar control and long-term weight control. Consider adding a daily fiber supplement to your Sierras Solution program.

EAT YOUR CALORIES, DON'T DRINK THEM

Sugared beverages contain no fat but are hugely problematic for weight controllers. While the focus of Simple Change #1 is on fat, weight controllers also keep one eye on fruit juices and regular sodas. Some of our students consumed over 2,000 calories *per day* of these drinks before coming to AOS. What a shame it would be if your weight controller did all the work necessary to say good-bye to fat, only to derail her success by drinking thousands of calories.

In the Sierras Solution, we eat our calories. We don't drink them.

In one ten-week study, volunteers who drank regular sodas consumed an extra 500 to 700 calories a day and gained three and a half pounds; they also increased their blood pressure. Those who drank diet soda lost two pounds.

Diet soda can be a good beverage substitute, not only for regular soda but also for fruit juice. A study at Harvard University found that for each additional sugared drink (juice, soda, or sports drink) consumed by middle-school children, the risk of becoming obese increased by 60 percent. Even the American Academy of Pediatrics now recommends diet sodas over fruit juices for this reason. Fruit juice, even 100 percent fruit juice, provides almost no fiber and lots of concentrated sugary calories that increase the total calories consumed per day.

One major exception to the "Don't drink your calories" rule is fat-free milk. Fat-free milk contains good amounts of protein (9 grams per glass) and lots of calcium. Some research even shows that consuming lots of dairy products and calcium may help with weight control.

Please note: For those parents who are worried about the risks of sugar substitutes, please know that we hold children's safety as our sacred responsibility. We would never recommend anything we thought was unsafe.

The Role of Sugar Substitutes and Other "Nutritional Sacrifices"

For LTWCs, there is often no better friend than Splenda—a relatively new artificial sweetener that many weight controllers say tastes almost exactly like sugar but is calorie-free.

Some parents are concerned about sugar substitutes, including aspartame, which is used in most diet sodas. Some believe sugar substitutes are dangerous, even carcinogenic.

We believe there is a clear scientific consensus on the safety of many sugar substitutes, and we urge parents to consider the big picture. The FDA, the American Academy of Pediatrics, the American Diabetes Association, and even consumer protection organizations such as *Consumer Reports* and the Center for Science in the Public Interest (CSPI) have all agreed that sugar substitutes are safe; we think they are a very useful tool in helping to break the cycle of overweight in our kids. The following table was constructed based on CSPI's recent review of the safety of various sugar substitutes.

	ALSO KNOWN AS:	WHAT IS IT?	WHY IS IT LOW IN CALORIES?	SAFETY
Aspartame	Sweet 'N Low (blue packet), Equal, and NutraSweet.	A synthetic derivative of a combination of two amino acids, aspartic acid and phenylalanine.	Only tiny amounts of aspartame are needed to sweeten foods.	People who believe they suffer from headaches or other symptoms after consuming foods that contain aspartame might be wise to avoid this sweetener. However, CSPI concluded, based on the studies conducted on headaches related to aspartame, by saying, "Some people react to aspartame, though fewer than the number who believe they do." They also noted that there was no evidence supporting claims that aspartame "causes everything from Alzheimer's disease to multiple sclerosis." Only people with the rare disorder phenylketonuria (PKU), who can't metabolize phenylalanine, should avoid aspartame.
Cyclamate	Sucaryl, Sugar Twin, Sweet 'N Low (pink packet).	A synthetic chemical discovered in 1937 by a university student while trying to synthesize an antifever medication.	Most people can't metabolize cyclamate.	CSPI concluded that the better studies on this sweetener indicate that cyclamate doesn't cause cancer, but that it (or a by-product) appears to increase the potency of several carcinogens. Research in animals also suggests that cyclamate may damage the male reproductive organs. CSPI recommends avoiding cyclamate for these reasons.
Saccharin	Hermesetas.	A synthetic chemical.	Our bodies can't metabolize saccharin.	Some good studies do suggest that heavy use of saccharin may increase the risk of certain cancers, particularly bladder cancer. CSPI recommends avoiding saccharin for this reason.

	ALSO KNOWN AS:	WHAT IS IT?	WHY IS IT LOW IN CALORIES?	SAFETY
Stevia	Sweet leaf and honey leaf.	An extract from a shrub that grows in Brazil and Paraguay.	Our bodies can't metabolize stevia.	Even though stevia is a natural product (an extract from a shrub rather than a synthetic chemical), scientific evidence suggests that it could cause harm to reproductive processes in both males and females. The FDA and other organizations internationally concluded that stevia shouldn't be allowed in food. CSPI recommends against using stevia either in food or as a sugar additive for these reasons. They noted, "Stevia is promoted by the health-food industry as a natural alternative to synthetic sweeteners like saccharin, cyclamate and aspartame, but 'natural' doesn't automatically mean 'safe.'"
Sucralose	Splenda.	Sugar (sucrose) chemically combined with chlorine.	Our bodies can't burn sucralose for energy.	Sucralose passed all safety tests and animal studies. CSPI concluded, "There is no reason to suspect that sucralose causes any harm."
Sugar alcohols	Sorbitol, xylitol, mannitol, maltitol, lactitol, isomalt, erythritol, hydrogenated starch, and hydrolysates.	Sugar alcohols aren't sugar; they are made by adding hydrogen atoms to sugars. For example, adding hydrogen to glucose makes sorbitol.	Some sugar alcohols are not absorbed at all or largely unabsorbed, like erythritol, but others, such as maltitol, are absorbed enough to	Too much sugar alcohol can cause bloating, gas, diarrhea, and other problematic symptoms. The FDA requires a "laxative effect" warning notice on labels if consumers could ingest certain amounts during one day. The CSPI noted that, while sugar alcohols may have minimal effect on your blood sugar, they may have more than a minimal effect on your waistline and hips. In other words, the most commonly used sugar alcohols contain a fair number of calories and,

(continued)

	ALSO KNOWN AS:	WHAT IS IT?	WHY IS IT LOW IN CALORIES?	SAFETY
Sugar alcohols (cont.)			provide three-quarters of the calories of sugar.	therefore, are not good alternatives compared to products like sucralose (Splenda) or aspartame for weight controllers.
Tagatose	Naturlose.	A form of sugar that is manufactured from milk (lactose).	Most of this product passes through our bodies without being absorbed.	Consuming large amounts can cause colic (in babies), flatulence, bloating, and nausea. Animal and human studies, however, have raised no safety concerns beyond those unfortunate symptoms.

In the Sierras Solution diet sodas are "uncontrolled," and weight controllers may have unlimited access to them. We do post signs around the dining halls noting that diet sodas with caffeine can dehydrate you, and that the best way to quench thirst and stay hydrated is to drink noncaffeinated diet sodas, teas, Crystal Light, and water. But we don't fight a battle against diet soda or sugar substitutes in general. In fact, many other foods on the meal plan, including our many wonderful fat-free desserts, include various sugar substitutes.

When parents ask us about our use of sugar substitutes, we hear the same kind of arguments that we do about the benefits of a 100 percent vegetarian diet, or organic foods. Why don't you encourage vegetarian or organic eating? Aren't these healthier ways to eat?

We answer by saying, "We don't let the best be the enemy of the good." We believe the greatest immediate danger to the lives of overweight kids is the excess weight they carry. Although it might be healthiest to limit some diet sodas and sugar substitutes, or eat only protein that comes from vegetable sources, or strive for less-processed foods, each of these steps would significantly reduce the likelihood that your weight controller would achieve Simple Change #1, eating less than 20 grams of fat per day. For the long-term psychological and physical health of our weight controllers, we focus on weight loss first. Once we are able to return our students to a normal weight range and provide them with the skills they need to be LTWCs, then we can have a discussion about dietary refinements. In the meantime, we don't let an ideal diet—but largely unenjoyable and therefore impractical for most teens—distract our focus from our goal.

Finding Lovable Foods That Love You Back

One of the biggest challenges about adopting Simple Change #1 concerns the type of food your weight controller likes to eat. We've discussed how the biology of an LTWC differs dramatically from that of a never-overweight person. We know that LTWCs will:

- feel a desire for food in response to a wide variety of situations.
- find it very difficult to put food aside once it is on their plates.
- have an almost limitless capacity to eat at almost all times.
- have very powerful biological responses (like extra salivation and insulin flow) to particularly appealing foods, such as freshly baked cookies or hot pizza.

Allison G., a twenty-year-old who has maintained her weight loss for over six months, tells a story that suggests the special type of hunger experienced by overweight and formerly overweight people:

I went into my mom's car and got out a packet of jelly and was sucking on it in our backyard. My mom caught me, but didn't really make a huge deal about it. I definitely remember that moment, though, especially since my mom brings it up to this day. She always wonders out loud if that's the moment she knew I had a problem with food.

These desires for foods won't seem familiar to most never-overweight people. Those without Allison's biology simply won't have a similar experience to share. And their parents certainly won't be reminding them about it fourteen years later.

To manage these supernormal desires for food, LTWCs and their parents must work harder to stay on track. Remarkably and fortunately, the very low fat-diet actually helps LTWCs stay on track by decreasing appetite and satisfying hunger better than any other approach.

One key is to make sure this approach to food is enjoyable. If it's not enjoyable, it's not sustainable. If it's not enjoyable, it's "a diet" rather than "your lifestyle." LTWCs still enjoy food; they just enjoy different foods than they used to. They eat interesting and appealing foods that work for them. We call this "finding lovable foods that love you back." When you first implement Simple Change #1, try to zero in on each of the five following aspects of food to help enhance the food's appeal, or lovability:

Taste. As you and your weight controller eat, identify the flavors of your food: is it sweet, salty, sour, or bitter? You'll accentuate the flavors the more you focus on them. Savor very low-fat foods by making yourself aware of each element of their taste.

Appearance. Try this trick from our culinary classes: when you and your weight controller prepare your own very low-fat food, try to think of the plate as a canvas and the food as the paint. Focus on arranging the colors in an attractive way to heighten the experience of eating.

Smell. Very low-fat foods often have more interesting spices than higher-fat foods and never smell greasy. Smells are not only fat-free but also calorie-free! Whether you're preparing to eat buffalo burgers or fat-free cheese enchiladas, encourage your weight controller to enjoy the smell of the food as you both prepare it.

Texture. Whether it's crunchy vegetables, popcorn, pretzels, cheesy quesadillas, or fresh, juicy strawberries cut up in a bowl of creamy fat-free yogurt, you'll enjoy a wide range of textures when you follow Simple Change #1 in the Sierras Solutions eating plan.

Belief. Finally, LTWCs learn to change their beliefs about very low-fat and healthful foods. Studies by Cornell University nutritionist Dr. Brian Wansink and others show that many people automatically downgrade the taste of foods believed to be healthier before even tasting them. In the Sierras Solution, we encourage you to find the lovable aspects of everything you and your weight controller eat, and to work toward believing new foods and spices can taste great.

Creating the Fat-Free Home

Weight controllers become accustomed to having a variety of low-fat and very low-fat foods and snacks readily available at home. One of the best ways you and your weight controller can get started on Simple Change #1 is to create a fat-free home.

Together with your weight controller, pick a day to go through each item in the pantry and refrigerator. If the item has more than a few grams of fat per serving, put it to the side—it doesn't belong in your house. If you can't bear to throw them all away, give them to a neighbor or a food pantry.

Once this is done, it's time to restock the kitchen. Check out the list of Sierras Solution staples on page 116, a list of "must-have" items for your pantry. Or, take the shopping list for Week 1 (see page 301) and head to the grocery store.

We can't emphasize enough how important it is to go all the way with this approach. Study after study has shown that when children receive options in cafeteria settings, they tend to pick the unhealthy ones. However, when they receive no such options, they do just fine. We see this at AOS every day: when provided with only healthy foods, students report very little hunger and a great deal of satisfaction. We routinely reassess this and we keep coming up with the same conclusion.

This approach can work beautifully in your home, but you must go all the way to creating a fat-free home to reap the benefits of healthy eating for the whole family. Even having a few higher-fat options available at home sends the following troublesome messages:

- High-fat foods are the good stuff.
- It's perfectly okay to deviate significantly from your plan occasionally.
- The adults in the house can't follow the Sierras Solution.

You want to show your weight controller that very healthy, very low-fat foods are just as good as regular-fat versions. Do regular-fat chips taste so much better than baked varieties? Certainly the higher-fat versions taste greasier and you may discern some difference in flavor, but, really, most overweight adults would argue that the difference in taste pales in comparison to the importance of helping your child maintain a healthy weight.

Give some thought to what retaining some high-fat foods communicates about the adults in the house: "I can't follow this program myself. It takes too much discipline and dedication. That's more than I can do."

Think about it this way—if your daughter had severe asthma, would you allow someone to blow cigarette smoke in her face? The sight of high-fat food affects your weight controller at a similarly biological level—please make sure your entire family understands and respects that. Remember, "Do as I say" doesn't work nearly as well as "Do as I do."

One caveat here concerns families with infants and toddlers. Your pediatrician would want you to maintain a bit more fat in your baby's diet. The good news is that baby food has little appeal to anyone other than babies. Just consult your pediatrician for the particulars on this, but ask specifically when the baby can join the rest of the family in this healthful, very low-fat diet.

Shopping the Sierras Solution Way

Very low-fat eating begins in grocery stores. Because of the nutrition information labels on almost every item, the grocery store is a huge library of facts for you and your weight controller. Plan on spending more time than usual there to become familiar with how many fat and fiber grams your favorite foods have. You will likely be very surprised! While you're shopping, try some of these suggestions to help teach you and your weight controller more about the best foods for your program.

Use the Sierras Solution shopping lists. For each of your first six weeks on the plan, we've created a simple shopping list for you to use. (See page 301

The Best Strategy for Stress Eaters

Is your weight controller an emotional eater? Actually, all of us are emotional eaters at least sometimes. When emotions get the best of your young weight controller (and she doesn't find something else to do that is distracting or absorbing), encourage her to *deviate quantitatively, not qualitatively*. In other words, focus on satisfying urges to overeat with very low-fat foods when stressed, and avoid high-fat foods at all costs. She'll find it much easier to get back on track if she eats several servings of fat-free chocolate pudding rather than one serving of high-fat chocolate ice cream.

Deviating qualitatively from the Sierras Solution—eating high-fat foods—is not merely a problem because of the additional fat grams and calories. More fundamentally, if your child eats high-fat foods when stressed, anxious, or upset, such foods become the preferred remedy for the blues. Remember: the goal is to ensure that high-fat foods become *less* desirable over time, not sources of comfort. You both want to start looking at pizza with regular-fat mozzarella cheese as greasy and a bit disgusting. You want full-fat chocolate to seem too rich.

This may mean eating several bowls of fat-free strawberry yogurt, several pears or apples, lots of grapes, a bag or two of air-popped popcorn—anything but high-fat foods. And as a parent, part of your job is to keep lots of these foods readily available at all times. Many of these foods are what we call "uncontrolled foods" at AOS. For a list of our uncontrolled foods, see page 124.

Sometimes I binge eat on very low-density foods. Salad and fruit and vegetables can help me. For my binge, I'll usually do blueberries or something small like that. I just keep picking at it and eventually I get it into my head, "Hey, you're eating a lot. Stop."

—ALISON S., THIRTEEN, BEDFORD, NEW YORK
   INITIAL WEIGHT LOSS: FIFTY POUNDS IN FIVE MONTHS
   SUSTAINED WEIGHT LOSS: FORTY-SIX POUNDS FOR SIX MONTHS

Sierras Solution Staples for Every Kitchen

Spices, Condiments, Dressings, and Sauces

A1 sauce

Balsamic or apple cider vinegar

Baking powder

Barbecue sauce

Black pepper

Capers

Cayenne pepper

Chili powder

Crushed red pepper flakes

Curry powder

Dijon mustard

Dill pickles

Dried basil

Dried oregano

Dried rosemary

Dried thyme

Dry onion soup mix

Fat-free ginger dressing, such as Newman's Own

Fat-free mayonnaise

Garlic salt

Green taco sauce

Ground allspice

Ground cinnamon

Ground cumin

Honey mustard

Hot pepper vinegar

Ketchup

Malt vinegar

Marsala cooking wine

Mrs. Dash's seasonings (various)

Nonfat cooking spray

Nutmeg

Old Bay Seasoning

Paprika

Picante sauce

Pimentos

Instant ranch dressing mix

Red Hot sauce

Relish

Rice wine vinegar

Roasted red peppers

Salsa

Salt

Seasoning salt (preferably Lawry's)

Soy sauce

Spicy mustard

Splenda baking sugar

Splenda brown sugar

Splenda sugar

Tabasco sauce

Teriyaki sauce

Worcestershire sauce

Yellow mustard

Dairy

Egg Beaters

Fat-free American cheese

Fat-free buttermilk

Fat-free butter spray

Fat-free cheddar cheese

Fat-free cottage cheese

Fat-free cream cheese

Fat-free feta

Fat-free milk

Fat-free Parmesan or Romano

Fat-free plain yogurt

Fat-free ricotta cheese

Fat-free sour cream

Fat-free, sugar-free Cool Whip

Fat-free, sugar-free ice cream

Fat-free, sugar-free vanilla yogurt

Canned and Dry Goods

All-purpose flour

Angel food cake mix

Baked tortilla chips

Beef jerky

Brown rice

Canned fat-free beans

Canned fat-free soups (various)

Canned fruit in juice

Canned light tuna

Canned tomatoes— diced, sauce, paste

Canned vegetables

Caramel corn rice cakes (Quaker)

Chili lime chips, preferably Guiltless Gourmet

Crystal Light

Fat-free chicken or vegetable stock

Fat-free evaporated milk

Fat-free panko (Japanese breadcrumbs)

Fat-free pretzels

Fat-free refried beans

Fat-free tortillas, white and whole wheat

Fig Newmans

Green chilies

High-fiber, low-fat cereal, such as Special K, Corn Flakes, and Cheerios

Lay's Light fat-free potato chips

No Pudge brownie mix

Peanut Wonder— peanut butter substitute

Quick-cooking oats

Raisins

Sugar-free pudding mix

Tomato juice

Whole-wheat breadcrumbs

(continued)

Whole-wheat flour

Whole-wheat pasta—
angel hair, elbow
macaroni, manicotti
shells, etc.

Meats

Buffalo meat (lean,
97 percent meat to
3 percent fat)

Chicken breast,
boneless and
skinless

Lean deli meats—
chicken, ham, turkey

Lean fish—cod,
haddock, halibut,
mahimahi, snapper,
sole, tilapia

Pork tenderloin

Shrimp

Turkey (lean,
97 percent meat to
3 percent fat)

Turkey breast, roasted
and skinless

for Week One's shopping list.) If you've already completed the six weeks, or you're eager to branch out on your own, take along the Sierras Solutions Staples for Every Kitchen list (above).

Turn your trip into a scavenger hunt. Split up the list with your weight controller and see who can identify the best snacks and alternatives to foods like regular-fat pizza. You'll probably come up with some very creative ideas and have a lot of fun with these exercises.

Start in the produce aisle. Spend as much time among the fruits and vegetables as you can, looking at all the varieties. Make a pact to try a new vegetable a week—find something interesting in the store, bring it home and investigate a recipe, and experiment cooking with it with your weight controller. If you do this fun exercise once a week, you'll both have a wider repertoire in no time.

Choose products that help you. Frozen fat-free dinners, 100-calorie snack packs, and other fat-free or portion-controlled items can take out all the fat gram guesswork.

Eliminate impulse shopping. To avoid the many temptations of shopping in the market, check out online grocery delivery services, like www. peapod.com. and www.freshdirect.com (for New York).

Let your weight controller do the shopping. If your weight controller has a driver's license, he or she is ready for this responsibility. Once you've gone together a few times, allow him or her to do the shopping alone. Doing so will give him a great sense of ownership and responsibility for his plan.

Simple Change #1:
Eat Fewer Than
20 Grams of
Fat Every Day

—

Cooking the Sierras Solution Way

Some LTWCs become more interested in cooking as they learn to master the Sierras Solution. Some even become the primary cooks of the house. By following the six-week meal plans, you'll begin to learn many of the powerful Sierras Solution techniques that nearly eliminate the fat in your meals while greatly increasing the flavor. Try to be as flexible, open-minded, and adventurous in your cooking as possible—try new spices, methods, and ingredients. Don't immediately discount new takes on old favorites. To help guide you, check out some of the techniques below. You'll discover that you don't have to give up very much at all when you gain these skills.

REDUCING THE FAT IN MEATS

The best way to make sure you're staying as close to fat-free as possible when eating meat is to go with lean meats like chicken, turkey, and pork tenderloin, and lean fish such as tilapia and snapper. We also love lean buffalo meat: this red meat is a crowd-pleasing nutrition all-star, with a fraction of beef's fat. Luckily, all of these versatile meats can be prepared in thousands of ways—there's no reason to get bored.

Bake, broil, grill, or steam. All of these methods preserve the juiciness of the meat without adding extra, unneeded fat.

Use a rack. When roasting or grilling meat, place on a rack to allow the fat to drain. You'll be amazed at how much fat you used to eat unknowingly.

Get rid of the nonessentials. Always trim fats from meats before cooking.

Use marinades to tenderize lean cuts of meat, like pork loin and tenderloin, the white meat of turkey and chicken, and buffalo steaks. Make fat-free choices like red wine vinegar, juice, wine, soy sauce, and herbs. Marinate for at least an hour, preferably several hours.

Make extra. If you grill chicken or other lean meat over the weekend, prepare an extra batch, slice it, and refrigerate it for quick and easy meals later in the week.

Ditch the oil. Use vegetable oil cooking sprays, lemon or lime juice, or broth in place of oil whenever possible.

Skim your soups. Skim the fat from homemade soups by chilling and removing the fat layer that rises to the surface.

Use flavor-enhancing ingredients. Experiment wildly with herbs, spices, garlic, vinegar, ginger, mustard, lemon juice, wine, soy sauce, hot sauce, and salsa. (The recipes in the menu plan will give you lots of ideas.)

Develop a repertoire of quick, easy favorites. If you settle on a few standbys, you'll never be at a loss come dinnertime. Here are some suggestions for fast, low-fat chicken dishes that are sure to please everyone who likes chicken. You can substitute low-fat tofus, or pork tenderloin or buffalo steak if you like.

- *Sauté chicken and vegetables* with your choice of wine, herbs, vinegar, ginger, garlic, lemon, or soy sauce. Stuff them into a whole-wheat pita and add some fat-free cheese.
- *Bake a no-fuss chicken feast.* Wrap chicken breast, salsa, corn, and beans in foil and bake at 350°F for about 45 minutes (for several breasts), until the chicken turns uniformly white but is still soft to the touch. Serve with brown rice or on a whole-wheat tortilla.
- *Use warm chicken to top a salad.* Throw it into a mixing bowl with a lid along with fat-free dressing and tons of vegetables, and shake it up—this will distribute the dressing more evenly, which most people love.
- *Add chicken to whole-wheat pasta* with fat-free marinara sauce. Substitute some fresh, thin green beans for the pasta, for variety.
- *Break out the wok.* Stir-fried chicken and vegetables work really well with fat-free chicken broth, lemon or lime juice, or light soy sauce and garlic. Serve with brown rice.
- *Put chicken in the Crock-Pot.* In the morning, fill a Crock-Pot with chicken breast (or buffalo), your choice of vegetables, and seasoning—wine, herbs, juice, or soy sauce. Add enough liquid to make a soup. Turn it on and let it cook for about eight hours on the low setting.

LEARNING TO LOVE YOUR VEGETABLES

What a nutritional bargain vegetables are—high in fiber, virtually fat-free, packed with disease-fighting chemical compounds, and limitless in variety. Try some of these techniques to make cooking vegetables easy and delicious.

Get convenience produce. Many people fear vegetables because they dread the prep time. But vegetables come in so many ready-to-eat varieties. From baby carrots to preshredded coleslaw, options abound. Buy a large bag of green salad for one or two nights.

Squeeze on some lemon or lime or add pepper to steamed veggies—all highlight and enhance the flavor of vegetables nicely.

Make grilled kabobs using lean meat and vegetable chunks. Use your oven broiler if it's wintertime.

Top your tater. Add fat-free yogurt or sour cream to russet potatoes, or top with fat-free cheese and broccoli.

Char-grill vegetables right on the grill or wrap in foil. Cut a zucchini in half lengthwise and do the same for peppers, removing the seeds and stem. Add a little nonfat spray to the grill first and then grill the vegetables on high just long enough to char them a little. Turn a couple of times during the grilling.

Make fat-free chili with canned beans, diced tomatoes, and crumbled soy protein. Make a big batch on the weekends and freeze for snacks and meals throughout the week.

Try small sweet potatoes. They take about five minutes in the microwave. Serve them with fat-free, sugar-free vanilla yogurt and/or cinnamon. Sweet potatoes are also a great accompaniment to chicken or pork tenderloin dishes.

Round out a vegetarian meal with whole-grain toast and fat-free cheese.

HIGH-FIBER SNACKS

Here are some ideas to get more fiber from your snacks:

- Eat whole-grain toast with a slice of lean meat and mustard.
- Mix different kinds of dry cereal such as Kashi, Multi-Bran Chex, Fiber One, Bran Buds, or All-Bran for a tasty, granola-like snack.
- Try a fat-free dip with broccoli, green peppers, celery, carrots, or green beans. Make your own dip using dry ranch mix, dry onion soup mix, or any other dry fat-free seasoned mix and fat-free sour cream.

Sierras Solution Substitutions

In the Sierras Solution, there's no need to feel deprived—you can always find a delicious, easy substitution for your favorite food.

RECIPE CALLS FOR:	SUBSTITUTE:	COOKING TECHNIQUES AND OTHER TIPS
MEAT		Broil, boil, bake, grill, or poach meat. Choose lean cuts of meat and remove visible fat before cooking.
beef	buffalo, ostrich, emu	
ground beef	ground turkey, chicken, or buffalo	
chicken	boneless, skinless chicken breast	
canned tuna	water-packed tuna	
DAIRY		
whole-milk dairy products	fat-free dairy products	
regular cheese	fat-free cheese	
ricotta cheese	fat-free ricotta	
heavy cream	2 tablespoons flour plus 2 cups fat-free milk	
whipped cream	evaporated skim milk, chilled	
sour cream	fat-free sour cream	
mayonnaise	fat-free mayonnaise	
FATS/OILS		
butter or oil for baking	applesauce, puréed fruits (like prunes),	Use 1 cup of the substitution for every cup of butter or oil

(continued)

Sierras Solution Substitutions *(continued)*

Recipe calls for:	Substitute:	Cooking Techniques and Other Tips
	or puréed vegetables	in the recipe. It is better to use unsweetened applesauce. If sweetened applesauce is used, reduce the sugar or sweetener in the recipe by one-third. Puréed prunes work well in recipes with chocolate.
butter or oil for browning	nonstick spray, fat-free broth, wine, herbs, and seasonings	Use 3 tablespoons fat-free broth or wine for every 1 tablespoon butter or oil called for in the recipe.
VEGETABLES	Cook with herbs, lemon or lime juice, and fat-free broth instead of fat.	
EGGS		
1 whole egg	1½ large egg whites or ¼ cup Egg Beaters	

- Serve cut-up fresh fruit like apples, berries, oranges, peaches, and pears with fat-free yogurt or cottage cheese for dessert or a snack.
- Air-popped popcorn makes a great snack. Add seasonings—but not butter.
- Try fat-free string cheese and an apple.
- For a cold treat, eat frozen grapes or berries.

Quick and Easy Breakfast Ideas

These items may help you to create healthy breakfasts that you can grab when you don't have time to cook:

- High-fiber cereal such as Kashi, Multi-Bran Chex, raisin bran, Fiber One, Bran Buds, and All-Bran with skim milk and fresh or frozen fruit.
- Fat-free yogurt with fruit and/or high-fiber cereal.
- Whole-grain toast with reduced-sugar jam and fat-free cream cheese or fat-free ricotta, or half a banana mashed with cinnamon.
- Lean ham or turkey and fat-free cottage cheese or cheddar.
- Plain instant oatmeal or Kashi oatmeal with sliced banana and cinnamon.
- Fat-free cottage cheese with tomatoes or other fruit.
- Scrambled eggs made from fat-free egg whites, fat-free cheese, and vegetables (chopped the night before).
- 1 low-fat bran muffin. Make enough on the weekend for breakfast and snacks during the week.
- 1 or 2 low-fat pancakes or waffles served with fruit. Make enough on the weekend for breakfast and snacks during the week.
- Whole-wheat bagel with fat-free cream cheese (look for frozen brands with 210 calories per whole bagel, not the huge 6-ounce bagels, which can have 500 calories or more).

Restaurant Dining the Sierras Solution Way

We're eating out a lot more often—nearly twice as much as we did a generation ago. When we eat out, we are giving up control over the ingredients, method of preparation, and portion size. We also don't control the atmosphere, which often can lull you and your more vulnerable weight controller into making problematic food choices. Accordingly, restaurants can present the greatest challenge to weight controllers. But they can also lead to tremendous confidence—after all, to paraphrase Sinatra, if you can make it there, you can make it anywhere. Once LTWCs have successfully

Simple Change #1:
Eat Fewer Than
20 Grams of
Fat Every Day

123

Uncontrolled Foods and Snacks

Asparagus

Baby carrots

Bananas, fresh or frozen

Berries, fresh or frozen

Broccoli

Cabbage

Cantaloupe

Celery

Cherry tomatoes

Cucumbers

Fat-free cottage cheese

Fat-free dressings and dips

Fat-free egg salad

Fat-free tuna salad

Fat-free yogurt

Grapes, fresh or frozen

Jicama

Lettuce (all kinds)

Pea pods

Peppers

Pickles

Pineapple

Radishes

Spinach

Sugar snap peas

Tomatoes

Vegetable soup

Watermelon

eaten out a few times and remained on the program, they tend to pride themselves on always being able to find something low in fat to eat.

Try emphasizing the following points to your weight controller:

- It is your right to request that the food you order at a restaurant be prepared according to your wishes—your right to get what you pay for.
- Most restaurateurs want to accommodate their patrons. In a recent survey conducted by MasterCard, more than 90 percent of restaurateurs said that they preferred hearing complaints about orders directly. They want you to be satisfied and come back again and again.
- Some servers might resist providing you with the information you want about food preparation. Remind yourself of your right to this information. Then, try making a polite request, even repeated requests, if necessary.

This approach will work well most of the time. Here's an interaction familiar to most AOS alumni:

Patron: I'll take the chicken with broccoli and new potatoes. How is that prepared?

Server: How is what prepared?

Patron: The chicken.

Server: I think it's broiled.

Patron: In other words, it might be sautéed instead of broiled?

Server: Yeah.

Patron: Could you check on that for me, please?

Server: Okay.

(*Server leaves for two minutes to check on preparation of the chicken and then returns.*)

Server: It's broiled.

Patron: Great. Then I'll go with the chicken. I'd like the vegetables grilled, with no butter added on them.

Server: I don't think they put any butter on the vegetables or the potatoes.

Patron: Please be sure that no butter or any sauces are added to the broccoli or the potatoes, okay?

Server: Okay.

Does this patron seem overly pushy to you? If you or your weight controller answered yes, you might benefit from additional work on managing this high-risk situation. Try explaining to your child that getting what you pay for includes knowing what you're getting. If your server does not comply with reasonable requests for this kind of information, you could ask to speak to the manager or the owner. You could also leave the restaurant. Staying at a restaurant and eating foods you want to avoid simply does not work for LTWCs.

Simple Change #1:
Eat Fewer Than
20 Grams of
Fat Every Day

———

A critical thing to remember when ordering in restaurants is, *If you don't know what the food is or how it was prepared, assume the worst!* This saying directs you to find something on the menu you can rely on. If you look diligently enough, you, too, can almost always find something to eat, no matter how challenging the menu.

MODELING IN RESTAURANTS

A family on the Sierras Solution plan knows that modeling in restaurants means *all* family members order in a similar style. The rationale for this is the same as when creating the fat-free home—it's unhelpful and unfair if family members order, and thereby endorse, high-fat, problematic foods in front of your weight controller.

Consider how you might respond in the following situation after you've settled in with your daughter at a comfortable restaurant for what was supposed to be a pleasant dinner.

> Mother: So, what are you all thinking of ordering?
> Daughter: I've been doing so well on my program, I've decided I want to get a cheeseburger and french fries tonight.
> Mother: Well, you know that seems kind of self-destructive, doesn't it?
> Daughter: Well, not really. I'll self-monitor it. Nobody does the Sierras Solution perfectly. You know that.

Most parents find this situation troublesome and have difficulty coming up with a good solution. At AOS, we recommend the following to parents, even though it might seem like a rather hard line to take:

Agree as a family, before going out to eat, that everyone will follow the Sierras Solution at home and when they eat out at a restaurant. Have a discussion about this, but get a commitment from everyone who will be eating in the restaurant before you leave the house.

If any child, including the weight controller, decides to order a food that's inconsistent with the Sierras Solution, then the parent will take the following stance:

1. Parents will not pay for such food.
2. Even if the child decides to pay for it himself, parents will not allow him to sit with the family during that meal.

Challenging Cuisines—Suggestions for Very Low-Fat Meals

LTWCs often lament limited choices in certain types of restaurants, particularly Mexican and Chinese. Small-town diners offer their own set of challenges. Still, some AOS alumni pride themselves on always being able to find something to eat. Here's a list of challenging cuisines and some suggestions from AOS alumni:

- **Cajun.** Seafood or vegetable gumbo or jambalaya (without sausage), grilled fish.
- **Chinese.** First, ask what can be prepared without oil. Try stir-fries prepared with fat-free sauces, broths, or soy sauce; chicken, seafood, and vegetables; soups (hot and sour, chicken, vegetable); chicken and shrimp dishes steamed without sauces.
- **Diners.** Chicken dinner (grilled or broiled) with baked potato and steamed mixed vegetables. If there's a vegetarian special, order it prepared without butter or oil.
- **French.** Poached, grilled, or steamed fish; chicken and wine sauce; Niçoise salads without oil.
- **Greek.** Chicken and fish shish kebabs; salads, couscous, rice.
- **Indian.** Tandoori chicken, prawns, fish.
- **Italian.** Pasta with red clam sauce; meatless marinara without oil; pizza with no cheese and with steamed-vegetable toppings; minestrone soup made without butter.
- **Japanese.** Chicken and fish teriyaki, sushi, tofu and vegetables. Avoid avocado, mayonnaise, eel, and mackerel.
- **Mexican.** Chicken and seafood enchiladas with no cheese or sour cream; tamales with no cheese; chicken or shrimp fajitas without sour cream or guacamole and made with as little oil as possible; and chicken taco salad (no cheese). When ordering salsa, ask for tortillas instead of chips to dip into salsa.
- **Thai.** First, ask what can be prepared without oil. Then, stir-fried shrimp, chicken, and vegetable dishes can work for you. Also try soups, especially sweet and sour (tom yum) soup, as well as chicken and cucumber salads.

Secrets of Successful Weight Controllers

Successful LTWCs invariably manage to consume much less fat than average Americans. Here is what this means in practice:

- They rarely eat red meat.
- They hardly ever eat desserts other than fruit or low-fat/no-fat alternatives.
- They almost never eat fried foods.
- Their salad dressings are almost always fat-free, low-fat, and low-calorie.
- When they order salads in restaurants, they ask for salad dressings on the side.
- They grill and broil and bake and steam foods.
- When eating out, they insist on being served foods prepared in those low-fat ways.
- They choose restaurants based on the availability of low-fat foods there.
- They rarely eat anything with high-fat gravies or sauces.
- They opt for fat-free cheeses, ice cream, and mayonnaise over the regular-fat or even low-fat alternatives.
- They take healthy alternatives to places where there may not be healthy foods, such as holiday parties.
- They plan their meals and even create lists of their common binge foods and brainstorm substitutions ahead of time.
- They think of normal-fat cookies, brownies, cakes, and candies as foods for others, not for themselves.
- They remind themselves of their compromised biology and know that these choices support their unusual physiology and long-term goals.

This approach means that if a sibling makes an issue of ordering a cheeseburger and french fries, you will ask her to both pay for the meal and eat at a different table alone. In our experience, no family has had to do this more than once. One dose of this usually does it. In fact, very few families have to get to this point.

You've learned all about Simple Change #1. You're bound and determined to strip all fat from your diet, no holds barred. But the food that goes in is only half of the weight-loss equation. Now we have to work on how that food gets used up as fuel. You're ready to add activity into your Sierras Solution program. Let's take a look at Simple Change #2.

Chapter 8

Simple Change #2: Take at Least Ten Thousand Steps Every Day

The single greatest predictor of long-term success in weight control is activity level. But most people in North America do not get nearly enough activity to produce many of the health, emotional, or other pleasurable benefits of exercise.

You and your weight controller don't need to run a marathon or spend hours in the gym to reap tremendous rewards. You simply have to put one foot in front of the other more often—each day, every day—and those individual steps will start to add up to Simple Change #2's magic number: ten thousand steps.

Scientists from around the world agree that taking a total of ten thousand steps or more every day is one of the most reliable ways to bolster your body's ability to shed pounds and lose fat. Yet, despite the fact that we all take thousands of steps every day, very few people have any idea what ten thousand steps look or feel like.

Depending on your stride, walking one mile is usually two thousand to twenty-five hundred steps. Taking ten thousand steps means moving four to five miles per day on your own two feet. Before your teen has a heart attack—five miles a day!—please share the good news that she is not starting from zero. The average North American gets four thousand steps per day—or walks two miles—just from moving around, walking from class to class, puttering around the house, and so on.

The difference is that extra six thousand steps per day—and those steps are directly linked to extra pounds lost. Those six thousand steps equal about an hour of additional walking each day—even less time if you move your body faster.

We know that getting in that extra hour of activity each day may not be easy all the time. But you don't have to do it all at once. Every step counts. Once you and your weight controller learn how to sneak in steps at every opportunity, you'll likely start to collect them steadily and meet that goal more easily than you might suspect.

The Benefits of Ten-Thousand-Plus Steps a Day

Activity can:

- Increase weight loss
- Improve maintenance of weight loss
- Improve stress management
- Improve quality of sleep
- Improve digestion
- Enhance self-esteem
- Improve resistance to illness
- Increase energy levels
- Reduce blood pressure
- Increase flexibility
- Increase metabolic rate
- Build strength
- Decrease depression
- Increase endorphins—the internally produced opiates that improve feelings of well-being and mood
- Decrease appetite
- Increase life span

Perhaps the most remarkable thing about Simple Change #2 is that weight controllers don't have to "exercise" in the traditionally sweaty and breathless sense in order to get the benefits of weight loss. Studies reveal that this simple, easy-to-fit-in activity is the preferred choice among the successful LTWCs who participated in the National Weight Control Registry. These LTWCs average one hour of brisk walking per day.

Check out this graph to show you the power of activity for long-term weight control.

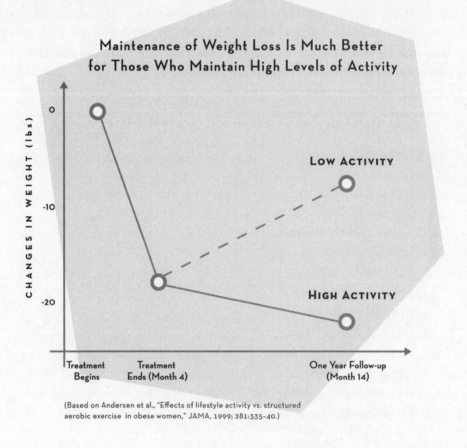

Maintenance of Weight Loss Is Much Better for Those Who Maintain High Levels of Activity

(Based on Andersen et al., "Effects of lifestyle activity vs. structured aerobic exercise in obese women," JAMA, 1999; 281:335–40.)

In this study, researchers from Johns Hopkins followed thirty-three overweight women through sixteen weeks of a structured weight-loss treatment program and then for one year after the program ended. The women lost an average of eighteen pounds during treatment, and you can see from the graph what happened after that. The group that exercised the most fared far better than the least-active group. This more-active group followed the study's guidelines to get at least thirty minutes of activity per day at least five out of the seven days of the week. They hit this goal about 80 percent of the time during the year of the follow-up. The least-active third in the study achieved that goal less than 20 percent of the time, and you can see what happened—they gained back more than half the weight they'd originally lost.

The best thing about Simple Change #2 is it doesn't require a gym membership or a nearby club or sports team—you just need to put one foot in front of the other. But some wonder if walking really is exercise, and whether is it enough. And what about the "every day" part—aren't people supposed to have a rest day?

To answer these important questions, we relied on a group of the world's leading experts on activity, the American College of Sports Medicine (ACSM). We've used the ACSM recommendations about the frequency, intensity, duration, variety, and strength-training requirements of exercise to help us make recommendations to you about Simple Change #2.

FREQUENCY OF ACTIVITY

The Sierras Solution goal is ten thousand steps every day. Not every other day or even six days a week. Every single day. Consistency is critical for many reasons.

Daily activity helps prevent the "desert island effect." When weight controllers reduce food intake and lose weight, the body reacts by lowering the metabolic rate. The metabolic rate is the amount of energy our bodies expend to keep us alive at rest. It includes energy to keep the heart pumping and the liver working to break down the food we eat and transfer the energy from the food into our cells. Even active people expend more energy on these bodily functions operating twenty-four hours (86,400 seconds) per day than they expend for movement and exercise. So metabolic rate matters a great deal.

When the body detects a reduction in food intake, it "thinks" something like *"Uh-oh, I've got to conserve energy to keep this person alive."* Remember, humans survived as hunter-gatherers for tens of thousands of years, and evolution caused our bodies to adapt by lowering our metabolic rate

> *The most challenging situation for me after leaving AOS was getting into a rut about movement. I'd make excuses and go back to old habits, like procrastinating by saying, "I'll go to the gym tomorrow." "I'll go walking whenever." Just making sure that I'm very consistent really helps.*
>
> —Allison G., twenty,
> Wichita, Kansas
> Initial weight loss:
> seventy-five pounds in six months
> Sustained weight loss:
> eighty-four pounds for six
> additional months

when we had trouble finding enough food. This "desert island effect" ensured that if you found yourself abandoned on a desert island, the metabolic shift might save your life by allowing you to survive on relatively few calories.

Staying active every day allows your weight controller to reverse the desert island effect. The first study on this, done in 1984, showed that about thirty minutes of brisk walking can keep the metabolic rate in a normal range despite lowered caloric intake of food. This finding has been confirmed in many studies over the past twenty years. Interestingly, our ability to reverse the desert island effect with activity lasts only about twenty-four hours. In other words, to keep the metabolic rate normal and make weight loss easier, weight controllers must stay active virtually every day, not just a few or even most days of the week.

Daily activity is also more routine and therefore harder to avoid. With a daily goal, it's hard to make excuses. This contrasts with a five-day-a-week goal, where most people will wind up saying to themselves: "Today is the day I won't exercise. I'll exercise tomorrow." This kind of thinking tends to result in skipping one day after another, and then abandonment.

Many AOS students find it useful to say to themselves: "Not moving is simply not an option." They remind themselves that their inner biological opponent never takes a day off either.

When I first got to AOS, I could barely walk. It took about two hundred pounds of weight loss until I could start getting involved with everybody at AOS a lot and then two hundred fifty pounds of weight loss until I could start running. I ran my last timed mile in less than ten minutes. And now I go to play street hockey every Sunday with a group of fellows.

—TERRY H., FIFTEEN,
EXETER, NEW HAMPHIRE
INITIAL WEIGHT LOSS:
305 POUNDS IN SIXTEEN MONTHS
SUSTAINED WEIGHT LOSS:
280 POUNDS FOR OVER ONE YEAR

INTENSITY OF ACTIVITY

Intensity refers to how hard your body works over a period of time. More intensive activity means the body works harder for the fifteen or thirty or forty-five minutes when you're active.

Intensity varies depending on one's level of conditioning or fitness. For example, world-class marathoners can run three eight-minute miles in a row without breaking a sweat. To the average person, this intensity would prove extremely challenging.

Many new AOS students make the mistake of exercising too intensely for their current fitness levels. As a result, they become tired and find exercise painful after only a few minutes. This is one reason why we typically start every AOS student's activity program with morning walks at their own pace. Terry H. started in exactly this way. But at his original weight of 558 pounds, he found he couldn't walk very long without pain and exhaustion. So he went swimming instead. Other students begin by riding a bike because it places less strain on their knees. A chart at the end of this chapter, "Step Equivalents per Minute," shows the number of steps each minute you can count for swimming, biking, and other activities.

Just be sure that the intensity is low enough to achieve the ten thousand steps (or the equivalent in other activities). The most important rule of thumb about intensity is: Keep the intensity low enough to allow yourself to be active comfortably for at least thirty minutes per session. In this way, intensity has a direct impact on duration.

DURATION OF ACTIVITY

The American College of Sports Medicine endorses activity sessions lasting from thirty to sixty minutes. However, many overweight kids have difficulty maintaining aerobic activity for thirty minutes or more. If your weight controller has trouble, try starting with sessions that last ten or fifteen minutes. Two fifteen-minute sessions of exercise produce about the same benefits as one thirty-minute session. In fact, from a weight-control perspective, weight controllers enjoy better results with frequent exercise for shorter amounts of time than with one long session.

Some confusing theories exist about required duration of activity. One concerns "fat burning," suggesting you won't "burn fat" unless you're active for an extended period. This assertion is wrong. When you begin activity, you begin using calories immediately. Initially, the energy consumed by your body comes from glucose stored in the muscles. As you exercise for longer periods of time, your body begins dipping into its energy reserves (fat). However, your body must replenish the energy supply it uses. This means that when you consume energy in the form of stored glucose from the muscles, your body will use its stored energy supply to replenish the glucose taken from the muscles. It makes no difference whether you're active for short bursts of ten or fifteen minutes or for longer periods of thirty to sixty minutes per session. Both ways burn fat.

Duration is much more important than intensity for weight control. Consider how to get the most steps. If you walk for an hour, you'll get between six thousand and eight thousand steps. If you run as hard as you can for as long as you can and only go for five minutes, you'll get about one thousand steps. Most people don't like to do or just can't do such intense activities, but they can do lower-intensity things like walking for long periods of time. Keep this comparison in mind to remember that anything you can do to encourage movement of any kind works far better than promoting very intense activities that can prove frustrating and exhausting for overweight kids.

What Could Be More Simple Than Walking?

Walking is the most accessible and sustainable activity imaginable. Unlike most other forms of activity, which require preparation, transportation, and equipment, walking can be done at any time—even before breakfast.

We know that many overweight kids have negative associations with exercise. Maybe they've been picked last in gym class or have been cut from sports teams because of their weight. Maybe, like many of the kids at AOS, they've endured teasing during physical activity and thus prefer to avoid it altogether.

Walking allows kids who prefer a bit of privacy at the beginning to be entirely stealthy about their exercise. After all, everyone has to walk around on their own two legs. The simplicity of walking allows anyone to learn how easy it is to accumulate ten thousand steps without proclaiming to the world, "I am exercising!"

Also, the simplicity of the goal of ten thousand steps gives clear direction for what's expected of your weight controller. The goals are easily measured and the feedback readily available. Wearing a pedometer provides great feedback, not the least of which is that feeling it on your hip or looking at it over the course of the day helps remind weight controllers about their commitment.

BUYING PEDOMETERS

To get started with Simple Change #2, you will need to purchase a pedometer for your weight controller. Pedometers are remarkable devices that sit on your hip and count each step you take. Some cheaper pedometers (which cost less than $10) do this with a spring mechanism that may not measure steps accurately. The better pedometers involve a sensitive ball-like mechanism that moves up and down with your stride, as the elevation of your hip changes ever so slightly. You can get a more accurate pedometer for about $20, such as those made by Kenz, Accusplit, Yamax, and New Lifestyles (see www.accusplit.com and www.omronhealthcare.com). We purchase our pedometers through Accusplit and typically use the AE120XL model.

Rather than purchasing just one pedometer for your weight controller,

> *If I were to forget my pedometer one day, I would go back to my house to grab it. I'd feel really bad if I didn't reach at least ten thousand steps a day. If I don't reach this goal by near the end of the day, I just march in place until I get there.*
>
> —Terry H., fifteen,
>   Exeter, New Hampshire
>   Initial weight loss:
>   305 pounds in sixteen months
>   Sustained weight loss:
>   280 pounds for over one year

however, we recommend buying one for every member of the family. If everyone wears a pedometer, pedometers will feel more normal for your weight controller. We also find that siblings tend to get competitive about steps—and, in this case, a bit of rivalry is not bad for anybody!

Keep Gathering Those Ten-Thousand-Plus Steps a Day

Walking as a form of exercise is the definition of "sustainable"—name one other activity that people can do from age one to 101. As you start to incorporate the steps into your life, you'll fall in love with seeing all those digits collecting on your pedometer. The key to sticking with it is to wedge walking into everyday activities and find ways to keep it fun and fresh. Try some of these ideas, inspired by other LTWCs.

Join in the effort. As mentioned earlier, buy pedometers for the whole family and insist upon their usage. If you can take the time to be active with your child, you'll probably see major changes. The best way you can be a role model is to consistently achieve ten thousand steps per day—that will speak volumes about how much you value this goal. Post a chart on the refrigerator that allows all family members to record the number of steps walked each day. Many of our alumni use this very natural form of movement to create a more active lifestyle for their entire families.

Start with a timed mile. At AOS, when students first arrive, we have them walk or run a timed mile. At certain points during the program, they repeat it, and then they do one final timed mile before they finally leave the program and go home. Try this with your weight controller—go to a walking track with a measured mile and time each other. Then check back on a monthly or bi-monthly basis. Watching the seconds (and minutes!) drop as well as the pounds can be a tremendous confidence and motivation booster.

If your family wears pedometers, then all the better 'cause it's a lot easier to do it as a group activity. It's more normal and easier if you have a group of people around to do it with you.

—Lawrence M., fifteen,
 New York, New York
 Initial weight loss:
 ninety pounds in seven months
 Sustained weight loss:
 eighty-six pounds for over four
 months

Give your weight controller a movement soundtrack. Many young weight controllers enjoy walking a lot more if they can listen to music on their iPods. Walkers and runners actually move more and at higher intensities (faster) when listening to music.

Reinforce with extra rewards. Try using the purchase of a new iPod or MP3 player as a reward for a significant commitment to the program. You

The biggest help was that my mom was willing to get up with me at 6:00 a.m. before school. I asked her if she would go walking with me every morning and she did.

—Annya M., fourteen,
 Orosi, California
 Initial weight loss:
 151 pounds in nine months
 Sustained weight loss:
 193 pounds after six additional months

At AOS, my first timed mile was twenty-two minutes. The last timed mile I did was nine minutes forty-seven seconds. Exercise became a really important thing to me. I was always trying to improve. The first time I did that timed mile, I walked it. I thought that I couldn't run, but the truth is I just wouldn't run. Now, I'm in a gym membership and running and doing other things like that. I really want to join a sports team because it would be more fun to exercise that way instead of on my own.

—Allison G., twenty,
Wichita, Kansas
Initial weight loss:
seventy-five pounds in six months
Sustained weight loss:
eighty-four pounds for six additional months

might even create a reward system in which part of your weight controller's allowance is contingent upon reaching a step goal at least five days per week.

Model movement. As a weight controller yourself, walk instead of ride whenever possible. Park farther away from destinations to get some extra steps in your daily life. And you don't necessarily need to be active *with* your weight controller. Enrolling in new classes or taking up a sport yourself will communicate loud and clear the value you are placing on activity. Your household will see a subtle shift toward being more active.

Make vacations movement-oriented. Many cities are great walking destinations and full of attractions for wide ranges of interests and ages, such as New York City, Washington, D.C., and Boulder, Colorado. Long-distance or even local bike trips and hiking trips can be a tremendous bonding experience, as well as a great activity precedent.

Buy a treadmill and get your steps inside. We recommend treadmills because we've definitely seen that they're more likely to be used than the more strenuous elliptical trainers or other equipment. When you buy a treadmill, rather than choosing a relatively inexpensive home model from a consumer fitness company (which tend to break fairly easily and aren't particularly sturdy), try calling around to local gyms to see if they have any used commercial-grade treadmills they are looking to sell. Also look on www.ebay.com and www.craigslist.com. You're almost always better off with a used commercial-grade treadmill than a brand-new treadmill designed for the home market.

Walk while watching TV. Put the treadmill in the room where the most television is watched—either the living room, family room, or, in some cases, your child's bedroom. Position it directly in front of the TV, at just the right angle to block the view from where your weight controller most likes to sit. This way, the best viewing will be from the treadmill itself. And, of course, the best way you can encourage frequent use of this treadmill is to use it yourself when you watch television.

Remove TVs and even computers from your children's rooms. Your children will spend much less time watching and, by definition, more time being active. Once the TV is gone from his room, support your child's efforts to get in the steps by immediately relinquishing the family TV if he's interested in watching a show—just as long as he's walking at the same time, of course. Limit total TV and computer time to two hours per day.

Create walking opportunities to surround sedentary ones. Believe it or not, going to the movies can be active. If you park a mile away from the theater and walk, you'll get an additional five thousand steps—perhaps enough to get you to the ten thousand goal for that day. Using stairs instead of elevators is another good strategy.

Buy a dog. Some studies have found that just by adding a dog to your family, you could lose up to fourteen pounds in one year—dogs have to be walked!

Get up early. Early mornings are the only time of day we all can control. The rest of the day might get busy, but you and your weight controller can always control what time you get out of bed. Mornings before breakfast are

> *We don't drive around the parking lot looking for the closest parking spot. We just find, like, the first one, even if it's way back there.*
>
> —TAMARA B., SIXTEEN,
> KODIAK, ALASKA
> INITIAL WEIGHT LOSS:
> FIFTY-THREE POUNDS IN THREE MONTHS
> SUSTAINED WEIGHT LOSS:
> SEVENTY-FIVE POUNDS FOR OVER
> ONE YEAR

Simple Change #2:
Take at Least
Ten Thousand
Steps Every Day

———

141

the critical time to begin getting some steps. Even thirty minutes goes a long way toward the goal of ten thousand steps per day. Plan to wake up thirty minutes early to walk together.

Walk your errands. If you're lucky enough to have sidewalks or walkable streets in your town, use them. Walk to the bank, the library, the post office, even a restaurant. Allow your child to walk home from school if the way is protected from road traffic. Try to leave your car at home as much as possible. Make a game out of guessing the number of steps it takes to go from one place to another.

Getting Steps in Other Ways

You've heard the expression "Variety is the spice of life." So it is with getting your ten thousand steps, particularly when you first begin. Variety adds excitement and increases the likelihood that your weight controller will continue to achieve this important goal.

You and your weight controller can also add steps with other activities. See the Steps Equivalent per Minute chart on page 146 to find other ways of adding to your daily totals. Try some of these fun tips for working more activity—and more steps—into your daily quota.

Try a new activity. Provide active lessons for your children, including martial arts, fencing, yoga, or any sport that seems interesting to them, including ones that might not seem like "exercise," such as golf. Any activity breeds more activity.

Fill your yard with active toys. Put up badminton nets and basketball hoops. Challenge your weight controller to a nightly ten-minute game, before or after dinner. Get your kids a street-hockey net, soccer balls, baseball gloves—anything that encourages active outdoor play.

Sitting versus Standing versus Moving

Take a look at the differences in calorie burn between sitting or lying down versus standing quietly versus walking fast. Standing up expends 20 percent more energy than sitting down. Walking fast expends more than 300 percent more energy than sitting down.

Sitting or lying down	2.0 calories per minute
Standing quietly	2.4 calories per minute
Walking fast (4 mph)	8.2 calories per minute
Running (9 min. mile)	17.6 calories per minute

Even shopping expends almost three times more energy as sitting, as long as you keep moving. Some adult weight controllers even purchase desks that allow them to stand up (such as drafting tables) just to get that extra 20 percent energy expenditure. Start thinking about this motto: Don't sit when you can stand; don't stand when you can walk; don't walk when you can run. If you can help your weight controller see the accumulation of steps and the burning of calories as a good thing, you've just done a great deal to support her likelihood of long-term success.

Make family outings fun and active. Do "special" outings more often, always with an eye toward being more active together. Try bowling, miniature golf, a game of Frisbee at the park, set up a Ping-Pong table in the basement. Your child will see this time together as a tremendous show of love and support—and a lot of fun, too.

Don't forget about the arts. Acting in a school play keeps students from sitting and instant-messaging. It gets them involved with other people and requires a fair amount of movement. Many people love to get involved in different types of dancing, either under-eighteen clubs or more formal classes. Encourage those long-buried performance dreams to come out again.

Simple Change #2:
Take at Least
Ten Thousand
Steps Every Day

—

Sierras Solution Success Story—Alison S.

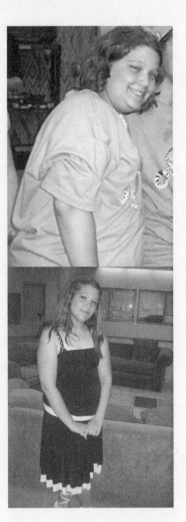

Alison grew up very close to her three sisters and parents. She remembers always being chubbier than everyone else. Throughout childhood, Alison loved ballet. The turning point came when she had to be checked out by a doctor to make sure she was strong enough to sustain her weight on her toes. Her doctor told her that her weight was such that she would crush her feet. Her desire to continue dancing is what pushed her to finally find a solution to her weight.

I didn't realize that it wasn't my weight that made others see me as untouchable. In fact, they saw me as an intelligent person. I created the idea that I was a loner when I withdrew from everyone. It was then that everyone began to see me as smart, but not much fun to be around.

My perspective on life did a complete 180 in middle school. I guess what sparked these changes was simply knowing too much. I became very cynical. Watching the news, I thought that human beings were just cruel creatures who were unable to live with each other and the rest of the world.

I started to slowly hate myself and wished I could just hurry up and die. I basically became very negative because I was growing up and I didn't want to. I did not want to think about my future, because I didn't want to experience it. I was pretending to be happy and okay when really I was slowly dying on the inside.

Since coming to AOS, I have little or no thoughts about hurting myself or dying because, for once in my life, I am truly happy. I'm loving myself for who

(continued)

I am and I am more comfortable with myself. I am starting to think about what motivates people to do things, both good and bad. When someone is mad or upset, I try to imagine how that person is thinking so I can be more accepting and comforting to him or her. I am becoming a positive influence. I have finally reached the point of true intelligence because now, not only am I book-smart, I'm life-smart. I am on my way to becoming an LTWC and I know how to keep myself emotionally okay.

—ALISON S., THIRTEEN, BEDFORD, NEW YORK
INITIAL WEIGHT LOSS: FIFTY POUNDS IN FIVE MONTHS
SUSTAINED WEIGHT LOSS: FORTY-SIX POUNDS FOR OVER SIX MONTHS

Make your yearly traditions daily ones. Does your family have a yearly game of touch football before your Thanksgiving feast? Great! How about a pickup game every night, or a walk, or a stroll with the puppy together? Creating these fun but predictable daily routines will slip lots of extra steps into your day.

Do everything, all the time, all at once. The more options your child has (such as the morning walk with Mom, basketball with brother, treadmill in front of the TV), the more likely the daily goal of at least ten thousand steps will be achieved. Every new chunk of activity is great, but don't stop with one—add new ones all the time, and keep adding. Some things will fall out, some will stick—better to have plenty to choose from than one that gets too stale.

Calculate the steps from other activities. Check out the chart below to see how many steps your weight controller's favorite activities will add to her daily total. If your daughter is trying to figure out how long she'll need to go roller skating in order to get the equivalent of ten thousand steps, the table shows that moderate roller-skating counts for 150 steps per minute. So after an hour and six minutes of roller-skating, she will have the equivalent of ten thousand steps.

Step Equivalents per Minute

ACTIVITY	EQUIVALENT NUMBER OF STEPS per MINUTE OF ACTIVITY
Aerobic dancing (low impact)	115
Aerobics (intense)	190
Aerobic step training (4-inch step)	145
Badminton	150
Basketball (leisurely, non-game)	130
Bicycling (5 mph)	55
Bicycling (10 mph)	125
Bicycling (12 mph)	200
Bowling	55
Canoeing (2.5 mph)	70
Cross-country skiing (fast)	330
Cross-country skiing (leisurely)	155
Cross-country skiing (moderate)	220
Dancing (fast)	175
Dancing (no contact)	100
Dancing (slow)	55
Elliptical machine (fast)	270
Elliptical machine (moderate)	200
Gardening (moderate)	90
Gardening (heavy)	155
Golfing (no cart)	100
Golfing (with cart)	70
Handball	230
Hiking (10-pound load)	180
Hiking (30-pound load)	235
Hiking (no load)	155
Housework	90
Ice skating (competitive)	170
Ice skating (leisurely)	95
Jogging (6 mph)	230
Judo (competitive)	185
Mopping	85

ACTIVITY	EQUIVALENT NUMBER OF STEPS per MINUTE OF ACTIVITY
Mowing the lawn	135
Racquetball	205
Roller skating (moderate)	150
Rowing (leisurely)	75
Rowing machine	180
Running (5 mph)	185
Running (8 mph)	305
Scuba diving	190
Scrubbing floor	140
Shopping	60
Shoveling snow	195
Skiing (downhill)	130
Skipping rope	285
Soccer (competitive)	195
Squash	205
Stair climbing	140
StairMaster	160
Swimming (25 yards/minute)	120
Swimming (50 yards/minute)	225
Swimming (75 yards/minute)	290
Table tennis	90
Tennis (doubles)	110
Tennis (singles)	160
Vacuuming	75
Volleyball game	120
Volleyball (leisurely)	70
Walking (3 mph)	80
Walking (4 mph)	100
Washing the car	75
Waterskiing	160
Waxing the car	100
Weight training (90 seconds b/w sets)	125
Window cleaning	75

Simple Change #2:
Take at Least
Ten Thousand
Steps Every Day

———

What About Strength Training?

LTWCs become runners, weight lifters, soccer players, martial artists, and many other things they could not have imagined before losing weight. All of these activities expend energy and most generate lots of steps—all except weight lifting. But don't let that fact stop you and your weight controller from looking into this very important aspect of fitness.

In 1990, the American College of Sports Medicine recognized and emphasized the importance of resistance training more than in any of their previous recommendations. Strength training of moderate intensity (50 to 60 percent of maximal lifting ability) provides important benefits. In particular, strength training can prevent injuries and help to reshape a body that's starting to shed its outer layer of fat. Many young weight controllers feel leaner, trimmer, and more empowered when they supplement Simple Change #2 with strength training. They also find they have greater muscular endurance for their growing portfolio of other fitness interests. While a weight controller need log only ten thousand steps a day to follow the Sierras Solution, strength training is an excellent addition to the program and can help you and your child see great gains in strength and endurance, in addition to many other health benefits.

SAFE GUIDELINES FOR WEIGHT LIFTING

ACSM's overall recommendations for strength training include selecting exercises that incorporate many different body parts and different kinds of movements. They suggest performing lifting exercises continuously, using smooth, slow, and controlled motions. Maintaining a good posture while lifting also helps avoid injury. Only the body part being exercised while lifting the weight should be in motion during a lift. Other body parts should be at rest and stationary during weight lifting. Here are some key guidelines to review before you or your weight lifter begins such a routine.

How many repetitions? Eight to twelve repetitions improve both strength and endurance. Most exercise experts suggest that if you can lift the weight easily more than twelve times, it is time to add more weight.

When you add more weight, go back to eight to twelve repetitions per exercise.

How many sets? The ACSM recommends using eight to ten different kinds of weight-lifting exercises per set. If you make time to do only one set, you will still strengthen your muscles 70 to 80 percent as much as you would by doing multiple sets. Two sets yields about 95 percent of the maximum benefit, and three sets creates the full benefit, or 100 percent. A full set of eight or ten lifting exercises, including warm-up time, can take as little as fifteen minutes to do.

How many workouts? The ideal strengthening program includes three workouts a week. Squeezing in more than three workouts per week might slow the growth of your muscles. Muscles may need some time off to recover from weight training. Interestingly, you can get about 75 percent of the maximum improvement available from weight lifting by working out only twice a week. If you don't have much time, even a single strengthening session per week helps far more than none at all. According to one study, a weekly workout can maintain current levels of strength for several months.

How much is enough? To keep building strength, you must keep increasing the weights you lift. You can maintain a desired level of strength by simply maintaining twelve repetitions for a particular exercise. If you stop weight lifting, your strength will begin to fade within two weeks. After three to five months, you'll be back to where you started.

PREVENT INJURIES AND MAXIMIZE BENEFITS

Several guidelines can help prevent injuries and maximize the benefits of weight lifting.

1. *Warm up* for a few minutes by walking briskly or jogging in place, and then do stretching exercises. It helps to stretch your shoulders, lower back, calves, and the fronts and backs of the thighs. Stretch slowly and steadily to the point of tension, not pain, and hold the position for three to thirty seconds.
2. *Breathe slowly and steadily* during weight lifting. Holding your breath while tensing muscles can cause light-headedness and even fainting.

Simple Change #2:
Take at Least
Ten Thousand
Steps Every Day

—

Exhale as you either lift the weight or raise your body, and inhale as you return to the starting position.

Perform the repetitions slowly. Each one should take about six seconds—two to lift and four to lower. Jerky movements can cause injury and soreness.

3. *Stop if your muscles hurt.* The dictum "No pain, no gain" is both wrong and potentially dangerous. Your muscles should feel fatigued during the last repetitions, but you should not feel sharp or piercing pain in your muscles. If you do feel pain, stop the exercise immediately.

4. *Cool down* after you exercise by doing a few minutes of walking or light jogging, followed by stretching again.

5. *Enlist a professional.* At least at first, it is also helpful for young people to have a qualified personal trainer so they can learn proper techniques and a range of weight-lifting exercises. A personal trainer should have a master's degree in physical education or exercise physiology as well as certification by the American Council on Exercise or American College of Sports Medicine.

Taking the Next Step: Planning

In appendix 4, you'll find a planning sheet that you and your weight controller can use to plan activities. We've included the following example, which was developed for AOS students to use to help plan their Thanksgiving breaks. Notice the level of detail and the fact that the students can choose which level of activity they wish to target.

As much as you might want to set the goals for your weight controller, you must realize that your child has the ultimate say in this process. For example, it's unrealistic to expect your child to completely give up the sedentary activities she enjoys. As long as she's getting more than ten thousand steps, she should continue to enjoy such activities.

The key is to focus on how your child will achieve the ten-thousand-steps goal—plan, encourage, and model. This can go a long way to promote the desired change.

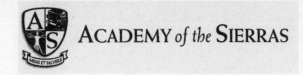

ACADEMY *of the* **SIERRAS**

Name: <u>Mary Sierras</u>   Date: <u>11/23/07</u>

Goals and Plans for the Thanksgiving Break

1. Steps per Day—Goals:
Minimum level: 10,000
Average: 15,000

PLANS:

- Morning iPod walk—45 minutes
- Walk the dog in the evening—20 minutes
- Pace around the house while I'm on the phone
- No escalators or elevators when shopping
- Park at the very edge of the parking lot and walk the perimeter before I go into the movies or the library
- Climb up and down the stairs while I'm waiting for dinner to be ready

2. Workout Activities—Goals:
Versa-Tube band every day—2/4 days workout

PLANS:

- YMCA with Mom at least once—try a yoga or Pilates class together?
- YMCA total at least twice—swim for half an hour, then do a half hour of weights
- Bands every morning

3. Minimizing Sedentary Behaviors—Goals:
Three hours per day max on TV and computer

PLANS:

- I'll walk to Cristina's house instead of calling her.
- I'll volunteer to shop for Mom.
- I'll ask the family to go bowling.
- I'll go window shopping/mall walking with Lisa.

4. Sources of Encouragement:

- I'll e-mail a friend at least once a day about how it's going.
- I'll bring Calorie King and read at least something in it every day.
- I'll look at old photo albums and see how far I've come.
- I'll talk to Mom and tell her what I've done every day and what I plan to do the next day.

5. Methods of Problem Solving:

- I'll self-monitor and write in my journal every day.
- I'll be honest with Mom and Dad and tell them how I really feel if I'm upset.

This planning sheet is a perfect example of how many different ways one weight controller can meet her daily goal of ten thousand steps. Her plans are specific and focused, which we've seen increases the likelihood of following through on them. This sheet also keeps Mary accountable to herself, which is one of the biggest reasons why Simple Change #3—Self-Monitoring—is so powerful. Let's look at that third and final Simple Change now.

Simple Change #2:
Take at Least
Ten Thousand
Steps Every Day

———

153

Chapter 9

Simple Change #3: Self-Monitor Every Day

A person who wishes to change himself should demand an account of himself with regard to the particular point which he has resolved to watch in order to correct himself and improve.

—Saint Ignatius Loyola

Saint Ignatius Loyola's thoughts on behavioral change date from the Middle Ages, but are still scientifically accurate today. Researchers have demonstrated the importance of self-monitoring—the systematic observation and recording of your own behaviors—to improve performance across a wide range of disciplines, including sports. Professional football players want to know how fast they run the forty-yard dash. Pitchers want know how fast they are pitching. Weight controllers are no different—many scientific studies have demonstrated the importance of self-monitoring for successful long-term weight control. Just as for elite-level athletes, self-generated feedback will help you improve your performance and develop the athlete's mental edge, what we call a "healthy obsession."

The Science of Self-Monitoring

We know this much: weight controllers who consistently self-monitor lose much more weight and keep it off longer than those who don't. No researcher or health-care professional who is familiar with the scientific literature on weight control would disagree with the value of self-monitoring.

We've contributed to the science of self-monitoring ourselves and studied results obtained by other researchers. Some results are astonishing. For example, weight controllers who discontinued self-monitoring during the holiday season (Thanksgiving to New Year's) gained 57 *times* more weight than their counterparts who continued to self-monitor consistently. (The weight controllers who self-monitored actually continued to lose weight.)

We believe that the magic threshold is 75 percent: when weight controllers write down at least 75 percent of their food intake and exercise, they are much more likely to be successful in losing weight and maintaining weight loss. Those who don't write down these critical bits of information have more trouble losing weight, and the pounds tend to reemerge.

At our Wellspring Camps, we found that campers who self-monitored most consistently during the four- to eight-week camp program were more than twice as likely as those who monitored less consistently to lose clinically significant amounts of weight during a six- to nine-month follow-up period. (See the chart below.)

We all strive to do better when we're being observed, whether by ourselves or someone else. In one study, Olympic-level figure skaters were left to train on their own. They were recorded attempting sixty elements (jumps, spins) in an hour of training. Then a whiteboard was brought out onto the ice so their coach could tally the number of jumps and spins in real time. The result: the number of elements attempted rose from sixty to one hundred. Then the whiteboard was removed, and the number declined to sixty. Then the coach brought the whiteboard out again. The result: suddenly the figure skaters were attempting one hundred elements again.

Don't we all, in our heart of hearts, want to get good grades? Just as these Olympians rise to the challenge, LTWCs know that weight control is also an athletic challenge. And self-monitoring is particularly applicable to this particular athletic challenge.

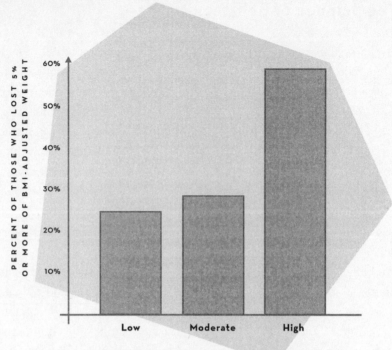

PERCENT OF THOSE WHO LOST 5% OR MORE OF BMI-ADJUSTED WEIGHT

CONSISTENCY OF SELF-MONITORING DURING CAMP

How to Begin Self-Monitoring

Each of the Simple Changes features its own basic tool that is instrumental for your evolution into LTWCs. The tool for Simple Change #1 is a nutrition fact-counting book, like *Calorie King* (as mentioned in chapter 7). The tool for Simple Change #2 is the trusty pedometer (as detailed in chapter 8). In Simple Change #3, you'll learn to use a tool that is perhaps the most basic, and certainly the most powerful, tool of the Sierras Solution plan—the self-monitoring journal.

Below you can see a snapshot of one page of AOS' Self-Monitoring Journal (or SMJ, for short). Pages from the AOS journal are also reproduced in appendix 5. We encourage you to take this book to a local copy shop, reproduce these pages, and have them bound into a nice little book.

We've created thousands of these over the years, and they've held the fine details of hundreds of fascinating tales of transformation. Start by dec-

Day:	Mon. Tues. Wed. Thurs. Fri. Sat. Sun.

Day: Mon. Tues. Wed. Thurs. Fri. Sat. Sun.

Date: _____

STEPS: _____ EXERCISE _____

Time	Food	Calories	Fat Grams
	TOTALS:		

MOVEMENT AND ACTIVITIES

Rating (0–100; 100 = goals reached + maximum effort):

THINK AND INK

LINK: _____

orating your journals with stickers, markers—anything to personalize the SMJ and establish more of a sense of identity and ownership.

HOW TO USE THE SELF-MONITORING JOURNAL

Once you have created your very own SMJ, filling out your complete daily SMJ sheet follows the exact same pattern each day.

1. At the beginning of each day, circle the day of the week and write down the date.
2. Starting with breakfast, write down *everything* you eat. This includes:
   - what you're eating
   - portion size (number of items, ounces, or cups)
   - calories
   - fat grams

Sierras Solution Success Story

Annya grew up in a small community in California's San Joaquin Valley. She remembers being overweight her entire life. Third grade was when other kids began teasing her and also when she started suffering from sleep apnea—a common serious respiratory condition in seriously overweight people.

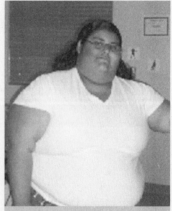

Since arriving at AOS with 407 pounds on her 5-foot, 2-inch frame, her sleep apnea is completely gone and she has cut the amount of time it takes her to walk or run a mile by 50 percent.

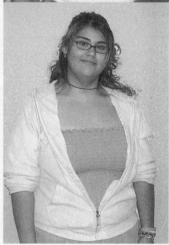

In elementary school I was really shy and didn't hang out with lots of friends. People used to make fun of me about my weight. I started getting heavy around first grade. When they made fun of me, I wouldn't protect myself. I was really nice and sweet. If people were new, I would say hi to them.

I got good grades when I was little. I was a little fat girl getting heavier and heavier. I didn't care if I got heavier. I couldn't do anything about it, such as run or play sports. In junior high school, kids would sometimes make fun of me behind my back. They would talk about me like they didn't know I was hearing them and I didn't have any feelings.

I had lots of problems with my weight. My parents and I couldn't really find clothes or shoes that fit me. My parents were getting worried. More kids started making fun of me. I struggled the most when I was in seventh grade because that's when lots of kids made fun of me.

(continued)

> *The biggest change in my life was coming to AOS. I was so happy to be there. When I was home for a few months, I first noticed that I wasn't moving very much and I gained two pounds. Once I realized that, I really knew that I needed to work out. So I just started going, going, and going. I went to the health club and I kept working out. The biggest help was that my mom was willing to get up with me at 6:00 a.m. before school. I asked her if she would go walking with me every morning and she did.*
>
> —ANNYA M., FOURTEEN, OROSI, CALIFORNIA
> INITIAL WEIGHT LOSS: 151 POUNDS IN NINE MONTHS
> SUSTAINED WEIGHT LOSS: 193 POUNDS AFTER SIX ADDITIONAL MONTHS

3. Repeat at lunch, dinner, and for any crumb of food that passes your lips.

4. At least once during the day, try to write down something—anything—that occurs to you in the Think and Ink section. (We'll discuss this in greater detail in chapter 10, page 179).

5. At the end of the day, record your total number of steps where it says "Steps" (top left).

6. Total your calories and fat grams for the day. Add them to the bottom of the sheet.

7. Review how active you were—on a scale of 1 to 100 (with 100 being you competing in an athletic event that pushed you to the limits of your capability and 1 being you lying in bed with the shades drawn watching TV), was today a 20 or an 80? Write that number in the "Rating" box.

8. Write your Link (we'll cover this more in chapter 10 on page 178).

How does this level of detail sound to you? If it seems like too much paperwork at the beginning, don't worry. Remember, don't let the best be the enemy of the good. In order to abide by the spirit of Simple Change #3, you can focus on two things:

Simple Change #3:
Self-Monitor
Every Day

---

1. ***Monitor fat grams:*** Note every bite of food that passes your lips and write out the food, amount, and fat grams, as shown in your nutrition fact-counting book (such as *Calorie King*).

2. ***Monitor steps:*** Check your pedometer, add any extra steps from other nonwalking activity, and total it up.

That's it. Simple Change #3 has been achieved for the day. You're self-monitoring.

Why Is Self-Monitoring So Important?

Many problems with weight begin when weight controllers stop paying attention. It's the hand in the chip bag, the endless stream of M&M's from the candy dish, the 20-ounce soda that was grabbed mindlessly. All of these carefree moments of consumption add up, often very quickly.

The Sierras Solution cuts directly to the chase by promoting consistent self-monitoring, the best way to keep aware of eating and activity patterns every day. When weight controllers self-monitor very consistently and observe the impact of their behaviors on weight over time, one concept emerges clearly: *everything counts*.

Weight control does not begin on a Monday or on the first day of a new month or on the first day of a new year. Weight control begins the very second a person makes a sincere effort to become aware of what she is eating and how she is moving, and she writes that observation down. Simple as that.

Self-monitoring shows weight controllers that even if they start the day with bacon and eggs and 28 grams of fat, they can still finish the day with very low-fat eating. Bacon and eggs do not contain an infinite number of fat grams.

When asked about how self-monitoring helped them, our students made some very perceptive observations about themselves (which is, itself, a skill strengthened by self-monitoring!):

- *Self-monitoring helps me stay mindful of what I'm eating.*—Lauren E.
- *Self-monitoring makes me knowledgeable about what I'm doing and keeps me linked to my goal of weight control.*—Tamara B.

> *Self-monitoring is the whole point of weight loss. You know exactly what's going in. Even if you're only eating what you're supposed to be eating, it's telling you maybe you shouldn't be having that much. When you see what you're eating, you know how to adjust it and say, "Maybe I shouldn't eat that," and whack it out.*
>
> —ALLISON G., TWENTY,
>   WICHITA, KANSAS
>   INITIAL WEIGHT LOSS: SEVENTY-FIVE POUNDS IN SIX MONTHS
>   SUSTAINED WEIGHT LOSS: EIGHTY-FOUR POUNDS FOR SIX ADDITIONAL MONTHS

- *Self-monitoring helps me solve problems and make adjustments in order to stay successful.*—Dan K.
- *Self-monitoring keeps me from feeling ashamed about what I eat. This helps keep some of the emotion out of eating and helps me stay more objective and focused on problem-solving in order to succeed.*—Courtney D.
- *Self-monitoring helps me cope, helps me feel in control.*—Lindsay S.
- *Keeping track of fat grams and steps in your head doesn't work nearly as well as self-monitoring on paper.*—Vicki M.
- *Self-monitoring helps you appreciate challenges like new restaurants. It is also the key to weight loss.*—Allison G.
- *Self-monitoring keeps me from lying to myself.*—Lauren S.

These LTWCs have identified most of the mechanisms that make self-monitoring the key to long-term weight control. Let's look at a few in detail.

STAYING CONNECTED

One important point is that self-monitoring connects the weight controller to the goal of weight loss, or as Tamara B. says, "*it keeps you linked to weight loss.*" It keeps the weight controller aware of the goal.

Let's say Tamara B. eats a medium-sized muffin that has 16 grams of fat.

The Sierras Solution goal for fat consumption is no more than 20 grams per day. Tamara has already eaten the muffin, but she has one more choice to make: she can choose to monitor that muffin, or not.

If Tamara fails to monitor, she distances herself from her goals instead of linking to them. Failing to self-monitor will probably lead her to ignore the problem and reduce her focus on fat grams for the rest of the day, and possibly longer.

If she monitors the muffin, Tamara is reminding herself of her goal of no more than 20 grams of fat per day. She is linking herself to her goal for fat grams and, ultimately, for weight control. As soon as she writes the number 16 in the column for fat grams, Tamara's motivation to limit fat consumption for the rest of the day will increase. Research shows that monitoring prompts you to evaluate how you're doing relative to a goal. That evaluation then makes you want to either keep doing well or try to improve your performance in order to meet the goal.

PREVENTING POOR DECISIONS

Like Tamara, most LTWCs won't skip the self-monitoring stage of this snack. It's not that they're not tempted by delicious muffins. It's that they're so committed to self-monitoring that the pleasure they might derive from eating the muffin is outweighed by the pain they will feel by writing the 16 grams of fat in their SMJ.

For most LTWCs, not monitoring is simply not an option. All Simple Change #3 asks is that you write it down. Simple—whatever they eat, they know they will write it down. Because they can predict how bad they'll feel when they stare at those numbers later, their ability to make a strong decision before they eat the muffin will be quite strong. They think about the pros and cons right there, in the moment—and because of that, are more likely to decide it's not worth it. In this way, self-monitoring reduces the number of poor decisions about eating.

ELIMINATING EMOTION

Most dieters think like this: *No, I shouldn't. I'm on a diet.* Then they find themselves trapped in a 2:00 p.m. meeting. They haven't had lunch, and there's a box of doughnuts on the table. They quickly scarf down two doughnuts while thinking: *I'm quitting this diet now. I'll start again next week, or maybe next month.*

Ironically, it's not the doughnuts that are going to cause them to regain whatever weight they've lost. It's what happens over the next week or next month. For most dieters, the doughnuts signal "Game On!" It's back to old eating habits until it's time to go on another diet.

This natural reaction is called the Abstinence Violation Effect (AVE). Weight controllers abandon their diets because they're ashamed about violating them; it is easier to abandon the diet than face the sense of failure for violating it.

Self-monitoring helps tame AVE, keeping weight controllers in problem-solving mode. Weight controllers who self-monitor focus on specifics—numbers, the goal, ideas for still meeting today's goal, or for meeting the goal tomorrow, even the act of writing it down. This helps weight controllers keep their heads in the game, rather than walking off the field.

WHAT AN SMJ CAN TELL YOU

Let's look at the SMJ of thirteen-year-old Alison S. (below), who has sustained her forty-six-pound weight loss for more than six months.

Day/Date: Thursday, March 7
Steps: 12,458

TIME	FOOD	CALORIES	FAT GRAMS
7:30 a.m.	Orange juice	130	0
Noon	2 fat-free yogurts	380	0
	8 garlic breadsticks	240	8.0
8:00 p.m.	4 small turkey sandwiches with Dijon mustard (on Hawaiian buns)	600	13.0
	1 bagel with cream cheese (reg.)	380	14.0
Totals:		1,630	35.0

Consider how it might have affected Alison S. to write this down. She recognized that the amount of fat she consumed on this day (35 grams) exceeded her goal of 20 grams per day by quite a bit. Writing it down ensured that she was thinking of the goal, which helped her renew her commitment to doing better the next day. On the other hand, Alison S. did meet her other goal of ten thousand steps per day.

Alison S. might also have realized that she neglected to eat any fruit or vegetables. Eating fiber would have kept her digestive system working efficiently. She also ate very little protein from the time she woke up until 8:00 p.m. This absence of fiber and protein may well have contributed to her lack of success in the evening. Alison S. rarely eats bagels with regular-fat cream cheese that have 14 grams of fat. On a more positive note, she chose turkey for her mini-sandwiches and, in terms of fat grams and calories, did quite well until the evening. She also walked her dog several times, in addition to shopping with her friends, to get some good steps in that day.

Simple Change #3 increases your commitment to focus on the details that help weight controllers keep going—even when they've eaten problematic food or when the scale doesn't cooperate. Remember: everything counts.

Take a look at Lauren S.'s first day at home after transitioning home from AOS (see next page). Although she had been nervous about how this change might affect her weight-loss efforts, on this day, Lauren S. met all three simple goals of the Sierras Solution. She ate far less than 20 fat grams, moved well beyond ten thousand steps, and self-monitored 100 percent of what she ate.

This is a great Simple Change #3 performance, although Lauren S. could have done better between breakfast and dinner in terms of nutrition. The SMJ is not perfectly filled out—note the omission of portion sizes in the evening—but it's pretty good. Lauren felt good about her performance as well. Self-monitoring helped her realize she could be successful in con-

Day/Date: Friday, January 13			
Steps: 15,075			
TIME	FOOD	CALORIES	FAT GRAMS
7:15 a.m.	3 egg whites	48	0
	1/2 banana	40	0
	1 slice cantaloupe	8	0
1:00 p.m.	coffee-bean drink	230	2
	chips	75	0
4:00–5:00 p.m.	3 Fig Newmans	180	0
	1 Popsicle	45	0
7:00 p.m.	ahi tuna	175	1.5
	baked potato	190	0
10:00 p.m.	frozen yogurt	240	0
Totals:		1,231	3.5

tinuing the Sierras Solution at home. This positive reinforcement and feeling of accomplishment may contribute as much to the success of long-term weight control as the value of the SMJ as a coping and problem-solving tool.

HOW TO MAKE SURE YOU SELF-MONITOR

As with the first two Simple Changes, some very simple strategies can help you increase the likelihood that you and your weight controller will continue to self-monitor. Try some of these tips to make it a fun experience for everyone.

Create SMJs for the whole family. Family involvement will help a lot here. If you can create an SMJ for every member of the family, your weight controller is more likely to monitor consistently. We know this from studying students after they transition home.

Initiate a self-monitoring after-dinner ritual. Self-monitoring together is a natural ending to the dinner meal, a way to keep the conversation going with a reticent teen, and a productive way to get closure on the day and

Q: Does It Matter How You Self-Monitor?

A: Not much. At AOS and Wellspring, we self-monitor in SMJs (as shown in appendix 5). When our students and campers return home, though, they continue monitoring online using our after-care website, www.myself monitoring.com. Fortunately, there are dozens of websites and software programs that do it the same way as well as various programs available for PDAs. The website www.calorieking.com offers software for your computer and PDA. Some weight controllers prefer to use a paper-based journal, others prefer technology. Regardless of how you do it, if your child begins to self-monitor very consistently, he will begin to do very well.

regroup for tomorrow. See it as a fun and collaborative experience, a way to help you connect as a family. You'll share better communication, helpful hints and suggestions, and maybe even some hard-won empathy.

Buy colorful, interesting journals or binder covers, and use fun art supplies to decorate them. Really "own" this book, as it will capture the most minute details of your very valiant efforts to change your life. Some LTWCs like to use their SMJs almost like a diary, including every thought. Others enjoy having a smaller, more discreet SMJ to take with them everywhere and just jot down the essentials quickly. Whatever works for you, do it.

Don't be afraid to get compulsive about self-monitoring. In times of high stress, some LTWCs find it very comforting to record all their thoughts about food. Others do better when they plan everything out first and then immediately self-monitor once the last bite is in their mouths. There is no one right way—like the other Simple Changes, this one is designed to be tailored to anyone's personality and lifestyle.

Perhaps the most secretly powerful benefit of Simple Change #3 is a trait it shares with the other Simple Changes—the clear pursuit of healthy extremes. With any of these Simple Changes, you might start on the modest side—but you can use them to go really, really big. Stay under 20 grams of fat a day, sure, but you're really trying to cut *all* fat. Reach ten thousand

My husband and I made a commitment to use the same tools, to monitor every day, monitor our activity, and eat the same kind of fat and calorie combinations. And we're still doing it. It's been seven months and it's great. What was really dramatic is how much it changed our understanding of Lindsay's experience. We went through some of the same things that she has gone through and will continue to go through, such as choices at parties and eating out. We've realized that part of the problem was we were contributing to her weight problem or weight-control issues by eating out so much.

—CINDY S., MOM OF LINDSAY S., SEVENTEEN,
 PALO ALTO, CALIFORNIA
 LINDSAY'S INITIAL WEIGHT LOSS:
 SEVENTY-FOUR POUNDS IN TWELVE MONTHS
 LINDSAY'S SUSTAINED WEIGHT LOSS:
 EIGHTY POUNDS AFTER ONE MONTH

steps, but strive to get *as many as you can*. Self-monitor just your fat grams and steps, or break down *every bit* of activity and *every bite* into your mouth.

Sound a bit obsessive? We hope so. We designed the three Simple Changes to lead directly to the development of a characteristic that all ultimately successful LTWCs share—what we call a "healthy obsession."

Chapter 10

Encourage a Healthy Obsession: Help Your Child Follow the Sierras Solution for Life

At AOS, we talk a lot about Lance Armstrong. Here is an athlete who overcame a true biological challenge—cancer—to win an unprecedented seven consecutive Tour de France titles. When a student resists getting out of bed for morning activity, the staff member will say, "What would Lance Armstrong do?" Lance's persistence was legendary, in one of the most grueling sports on earth. Here's what Lance says about persistence:

Pain is temporary. It may last a minute, or an hour, or a day, or a year, but eventually it will subside and something else will take its place. If I quit, however, it lasts forever.

Most parents know this intuitively: persistence wins in the end. But all parents have the same question: "Okay, now how do I generate this kind of commitment in my kids? How can we help create it or nurture it?"

This is exactly the purpose of the Sierras Solution's healthy obsession.*

*The healthy obsession concept and some other materials in this book appeared in D. S. Kirschenbaum's *The Healthy Obsession Program: Smart Weight Loss Instead of Low-Carb Lunacy* (Dallas: BenBella Books, 2006, reprinted with permission of this author and publisher).

Persistence is the key to helping your child follow the Sierras Solution for life. And nurturing her own healthy obsession will help your child develop a strong desire to change and persist, despite challenges every day.

The Healthy Obsession

Although the word "obsession" tends to have negative connotations in the outside world, at AOS we define a healthy obsession as "a sustained preoccupation with the planning and execution of target behaviors to reach a healthy goal." If an obsession is healthy, it will help you achieve a positive way of living. For weight controllers, a healthy obsession is a very strong drive toward achieving our three simple goals: eating a very low-fat diet, getting ten thousand steps per day or more, and self-monitoring. AOS students with healthy obsessions feel comfortable when they do these key things. However, when they don't or can't, they feel anxious, uncomfortable, or guilty.

Research suggests this type of single-minded focus can make the difference between fleeting and long-term weight loss. What finally helped many of the master weight controllers from the National Weight Control Registry to stop yo-yoing their weight up and down was simply a much more intensive approach. In fact, the majority of LTWCs in the National Weight Control Registry used in the final successful weight loss a much stricter dietary regimen (lower in fat), and more than 80 percent reported they exercised far more than in previous attempts. They also reported paying much more careful attention to their weight, their eating, and activity.

The three Simple Changes produce initial success. But it's the development of a healthy obsession that makes the approach sustainable and ultimately very successful. A healthy obsession results in more daydreams, plans, and routines that help maintain key behaviors. Remember, weight control is an athletic challenge—overcoming a biology that resists achievement of the goal. Also, our obesogenic culture makes it even harder to succeed. It's like trying to run a five-minute mile into a strong headwind. Our biology and the headwind never give us a break, nor do they give partial credit for moderate, albeit sincere, efforts. That's why it requires a great deal of persistence to become an LTWC. The healthy obsession, focusing the weight controller on consistency of eating, moving, and self-monitoring, will help LTWCs overcome these barriers to success.

A Healthy Obsession Is:

- Knowing that your biology has turned against you and does not cut you slack because you've had a rough day
- Accepting the tough goal of eating as little fat as possible every day
- Being unwilling or very reluctant to accept permission, even from yourself, to overindulge
- Accepting the idea that activity every day is the way, and doing it—even when you don't feel like it
- Knowing that "the devil is in the details" so that writing down all food eaten is vital
- Feeling anxious if the three simple goals are not met
- Understanding that everything counts—everything

A Healthy Obsession Is Not:

- Seeking moderation in all things
- Giving yourself permission to deviate from the program because of moods, stress, holidays, or vacations
- Waltzing into a high-risk situation (like a party or a Mexican restaurant) without a plan
- Making lame excuses for major lapses
- Allowing lapses to turn into relapses
- Feeling just fine when goals are sometimes not met

This heightened awareness starts with self-monitoring. By making everything count, self-monitoring helps create the foundation to the broader concept, the key attitude and approach, defined by the term "healthy obsession."

Using Bad Feelings for Good

The most successful LTWCs recognize they have a healthy obsession. They learn to hold themselves to a high standard of consistency for eating, activity, and self-monitoring. Their healthy obsessions keep them focused on the details and make them feel good when they achieve their goals, as well as anxious, unhappy, or guilty when they don't.

As you can see, a healthy obsession is much more than simple concern or worry. It is a dramatic emphasis on weight control as a part of a weight controller's life. If it is denied in some way on a particular day, the weight controller feels uncomfortable.

This discomfort actually provides powerful motivation to take action and fix the problem. In order to use that discomfort to effectively motivate change, we measure it with what's called a **Subjective Units of Discomfort (SUDS)** ratings scale, which helps students precisely describe the nature of their feelings. We use a 100-point rating scale to enable students to describe the intensity of their feelings in greater detail than they can with words alone. This scale ranges from 0 = no discomfort (relaxed or happy or peaceful) to 100 = extremely uncomfortable, miserable. Just putting a number to that specific feeling of discomfort serves two purposes— it makes the feeling that much more real, and it gives weight controllers another specific, measurable goal to improve upon their program.

LTWCs demand consistency from themselves in how they eat, how they move, and the degree to which they pay attention to the details through self-monitoring. Highly successful LTWCs do not make exceptions to this on a regular basis.

LTWCs do experience lapses—we all do. But their healthy obsessions ensure that the lapse isn't permanent and gets them back on track, typically quite quickly.

Helping Your Child Develop a Healthy Obsession

The good news is that after several weeks of consistently adhering to the three simple changes, the groundwork has been established. Your weight controller has probably experienced some weight loss and has a somewhat brighter attitude and mood.

But there are a number of steps you can take to help foster the development of the healthy obsession in your new weight controller. Let's review these according to each of the three simple goals.

Encourage a Healthy Obsession: Help Your Child Follow the Sierras Solution for Life

———

If I'm monitoring 70 percent or more of the time, I'd be feeling pretty good (about 5 SUDS). I don't get so worked up if I eat an occasional high-fat item because I can make up for it the next day. I do think about everything I eat along these lines, but that doesn't keep me from loving food just as much as I ever did (which is a whole lot).

—Terry H., fifteen,
  Exeter, New Hempshire
  Initial weight loss:
  305 pounds in sixteen months
  Sustained weight loss:
  280 pounds for over one year

Using the SUDS scale, if I ate more than 20 fat grams in a day, my rating would be 100. I would be miserable. Even if I ate one item that had 10 or 15 fat grams in it, my rating would be 100. I just don't let myself do that. I just don't consider it an option. That's part of my healthy obsession.

—Tamara B., sixteen,
  Kodiak, Alaska
  Initial weight loss:
  fifty-three pounds in three months
  Sustained weight loss:
  seventy-five pounds for over one year

DEVELOPING A HEALTHY OBSESSION FOR FOOD

LTWCs learn to enjoy the taste, appearance, smell, and texture of very low-fat food. And after six weeks of eating very low-fat food such as the Sierras Solution menu items listed in chapters 11 and 12, any belief that very low-fat foods don't taste great should be old news.

A healthy obsession for very low-fat food means not only a strong commitment to the goal of staying under 20 grams of fat per day, but also a negative reaction if the goal is not met.

When she first came home from AOS, I didn't cook for, like, two, three weeks. She cooked everything. (AOS also taught her how to clean, which is a wonderful thing.) My other daughters still ask for Alison to cook their favorites. The last few weeks she's even been roasting the chicken for our Sabbath dinners. The favorites that she learned at AOS include a spaghetti and chicken dish and a lemon chicken dinner. I'll also buy pizza dough and Alison makes them into almost fat-free calzones; she uses a soy product instead of meat and fat-free cheese. That's another big favorite. She knows the exact fat grams in everything she cooks.

—CARYN, MOTHER OF ALISON S. THIRTEEN,
BEDFORD, NEW YORK
ALISON'S INITIAL WEIGHT LOSS:
FIFTY POUNDS IN FIVE MONTHS
ALISON'S SUSTAINED WEIGHT LOSS:
FORTY-SIX POUNDS FOR OVER SIX MONTHS

If I were to eat more than 20 fat grams, then I would be wicked panicky. I guess the next day I probably wouldn't eat very much.

—JILL R., FOURTEEN,
FITCHBURG, MASSACHUSETTS
INITIAL WEIGHT LOSS:
SEVENTY-SIX POUNDS IN NINE MONTHS
SUSTAINED WEIGHT LOSS:
EIGHTY POUNDS FOR OVER SIX MONTHS

In addition to the positive emotions associated with weight loss, the healthy obsession creates a negative emotional reaction that inspires change. These negative reactions help LTWCs like Jill make better decisions and actions. Help your weight controller to understand that negative reactions like these are okay as long as they don't produce extreme negativity or depressed moods. LTWCs learn that feeling unhappy about violating the Sierras Solution's three simple goals can help them take action to get rid of those feelings. Overall, you'll see your weight controller's healthy obsession about very low-fat eating reveal itself in the following ways:

- Anxiety or other unhappy reactions when the three simple goals of the Sierras Solution are not met
- A major change in attitude about food such that food becomes something to monitor systematically instead of just something to eat
- A source of pride for eating in this way and acknowledgment by supportive friends and family members
- A new or renewed interest in cooking, modifying the content of cupboards in the household, and even cleaning up after meals

But developing a healthy obsession with food requires more than simply counting fat grams. It requires what we call calorie consciousness.

LTWCs become aware of calories. Eating foods that are very low in fat, high in fiber, and low in energy density helps control appetite and regulate weight. However, if you ate unlimited quantities of very low-fat, low-density, and high-fiber foods (two quarts of fat-free frozen yogurt, a couple of loaves of whole-wheat bread with jam on every slice, and several large bowls of fat-free chili), you would certainly gain weight. Allison G. realized that after she had mastered very low-fat eating, it made sense to start focusing more on her total caloric intake.

Critics of low-fat diets (typically boosters of low-carb and Atkins-type regimes) often point to the rise of low-fat foods in the 1980s and the fact that Americans have continued to gain more and more weight. These critics tend to blame the increased availability of low-fat foods for the continued weight gain. In fact, what has happened is that Americans have been eating about the same amount of fat in the past few decades, but we have also increased the total amount of food that we eat daily by about 200 (maybe even 400) calories.

LTWCs know that they have to watch what happens on the scale as they implement the Sierras Solution. If quantities of food go way up, regardless of the type of food, and activity levels remain low, weight gain will inevitably follow.

Although the eating plan and Simple Change #1 automatically help decrease consumption of calories, some degree of calorie consciousness is

Now, after having lost a substantial amount of weight and maintained the loss for a year, I don't focus mostly on fat grams anymore. I eat so little fat that the source of information that helps me the most now is calories. I concentrate more on calories to help me limit my total intake of food and pay attention to things like portion sizes.

—ALLISON G., TWENTY,
WICHITA, KANSAS
INITIAL WEIGHT LOSS:
SEVENTY-FIVE POUNDS IN SIX MONTHS
SUSTAINED WEIGHT LOSS:
EIGHTY-FOUR POUNDS FOR SIX ADDITIONAL MONTHS

absolutely necessary to become a successful LTWC. Always keep in mind that the Sierras Solution focuses on fat first, not calories. But after the first six weeks, you and your weight controller will add an awareness of calories to your programs, especially if your weight loss slows down considerably or stops altogether. To do this, you could add your number of calories into your SMJ every day. But if you're not interested in the daunting task of counting calories, try the following option:

LTWCs consume no more than eight hundred calories at the biggest meal of the day. This suggestion works quite well and maintains that beautiful simplicity that is the centerpiece of the Sierras Solution. Having a calorie ceiling for your largest meal keeps your calorie consumption more proportionate throughout the day as well as lower overall, without having to count every calorie that goes into your mouth. This goal is especially useful when you're out for dinner. Many restaurants serve enormous portions that by themselves can greatly exceed 800 calories.

A 2004 report from the Centers for Disease Control shows why attention to calorie consumption matters. According to this report, over the last thirty years men have eaten 168 more calories daily than they did in 1971. They now eat, according to self-reports, approximately 2,600 calories a day. Women have consumed 335 more calories over these past thirty years or

I went to this Italian place and decided to order the pasta knowing that it had no fat and that the marinara sauce probably wasn't too bad. I was shocked to see that it came out in a boat. It couldn't fit on a regular plate. I asked how many cups were there and the server told me about six. That was 1,200 calories just for the pasta. I asked to have a smaller plate and then had them box the rest to take home. We had pasta dinners for a couple of days from the leftovers from just that one meal.

—Josh S., fifteen,
  Tucson, Arizona
  Initial weight loss:
  sixty-two pounds in five months
  Sustained weight loss:
  fifty-seven pounds for over one year

so, increasing their total calorie consumption to approximately 1,900 calories per day.

Most nutritionists would argue that these self-reports are probably even lower than reality. Dr. Susan Roberts of the Energy Metabolism Lab at Tufts University notes, "We're now at the point that more than six in ten Americans are either overweight or obese. We didn't get there on 1,900 to 2,600 calories per day. U.S. food supply data indicate we're eating considerably more."

LTWCs master restaurants. Restaurants are the biggest hurdle for most weight controllers, and for many LTWCs, staying on track at restaurants is the true mark of a healthy obsession.

Most LTWCs students remain committed to the Sierras Solution in restaurants and other very challenging food situations by following a few rules of thumb, which are the very definition of a healthy obsession with food. Please consider making them family-wide practices:

- Before going to any restaurant, consider and discuss potential and appropriate very low-fat items that will be available.
- Bring your fat/calorie counter with you when going out to eat.

Prior to AOS, I probably ordered something fried with lots of ranch dressing or something to make it even more fattening. Now when I go to restaurants, I'm very careful about ordering things and making sure to have them without cheese. I don't even like going out to eat that much because I hate not being able to control what they're cooking. I don't order elaborate things for that reason. I just order something simple that I know they can't mess up.

—TAMARA B., SIXTEEN
KODIAK, ALASKA
INITIAL WEIGHT LOSS:
FIFTY-THREE POUNDS IN THREE MONTHS
SUSTAINED WEIGHT LOSS:
SEVENTY-FIVE POUNDS FOR OVER ONE YEAR

- Assert yourself about the method of preparation, even if this means asking for the food to be presented more than once before you're satisfied.
- Remember that the server and the restaurant are there to please you, and get you what you ordered in the way you ordered it. A healthy obsession for very low-fat eating indicates you're making every reasonable attempt to eat in this way.

DEVELOPING A HEALTHY OBSESSION FOR ACTIVITY

In chapter 8, the simple goal was to hit the ten-thousand-step mark every day, regardless of circumstances. A healthy obsession for activity goes beyond this important goal in two respects.

LTWCs feel discomfort when they're not active enough. A healthy obsession for activity means that your LTWC will feel uncomfortable when his activity goals are not achieved. Many LTWCs will walk in place in front of the television at 11:00 p.m. to hit ten thousand steps before heading to bed. It just makes them feel better. Some tell us they wouldn't be able to sleep well otherwise.

LTWCs manage weight through activity level. The second feature of a healthy obsession for activity is the management of weight through activity level. Henry E., sixteen, who has sustained a 108-pound weight loss for more than a year and a half, is an excellent example of this healthy obsession for activity:

With my weight, I'd say 210 is a very scary number for me. When I get to that number, I start exercising every day and eating terribly well every single day until I drive it back down.

When Henry sees a slight regain of weight, he becomes much more active, much more consistently, to reverse the trend.

HEALTHY OBSESSION FOR SELF-MONITORING

More than any other behavior, self-monitoring defines the essence of a healthy obsession. Consistent self-monitoring greatly increases your weight controller's smart thinking about weight control. LTWCs know that everything counts when it comes to eating. They learn to monitor every gram of fat. When those get too high, LTWCs cut back.

We've found that LTWCs' comments about their healthy obsessions feature self-monitoring, perhaps more than any other element. LTWCs know that self-monitoring helps them cope and focus on weight control. As with activity, some consciously use self-monitoring to manage their own feelings. It becomes a general coping strategy that helps them feel comfortable about their efforts at weight control. Others self-monitor as a means of improving performance, a tool that allows them to improve their focus on their eating and activity.

LTWCs start journaling. In the SMJs in appendix 5, you'll note that the right-hand side is a largely blank page with the heading "Think and Ink"

I love self-monitoring—it is such an important way of exercising control over my life. When I self-monitor, I can actually feel like I've done something good for myself.

—LINDSAY S., SEVENTEEN,
    PALO ALTO, CALIFORNIA
    INITIAL WEIGHT LOSS: 74 POUNDS IN TWELVE MONTHS
    SUSTAINED WEIGHT LOSS: 80 POUNDS AFTER ONE MONTH

Now if I'm starting to have trouble, like gaining some weight back, I monitor food, calories, the quantity, the fat, in everything. Monitoring keeps me aware of what I'm eating. I'll monitor until I get back to a good weight for me.

—DAN B., SEVENTEEN,
    MESA, ARIZONA
    INITIAL WEIGHT LOSS: 146 POUNDS IN TEN MONTHS
    SUSTAINED WEIGHT LOSS: 133 POUNDS FOR OVER 1½ YEARS

and another "Link." These sections are for what we call "journaling"—a variant on self-monitoring. In scientific research, the act of journaling has been linked to strong health results. In one particularly remarkable example, research on blood samples reveals that journal keepers have more active immune cells, implying better defenses against illness or disease.

Weight controllers can learn to maintain a journal in order to nurture their healthy obsession. Encourage them to write anything that comes to mind every day under "Think and Ink," preferably but not necessarily when they self-monitor (around mealtimes). We literally want them to put pen to paper and let it flow, without regard to grammar or focus. The "Link" section asks weight controllers to review what they wrote and note something of importance in this section—anything at all.

On the next page are a couple examples from Lauren S.'s journal. The first entry is from her second week at AOS. The second is from four months later, the first day that she returned home from AOS.

Two Examples of Lauren S.'s Journal Entries

9/10/05

Think and Ink

I can't wait to talk to my parents! They come in twenty days! I am really excited! On my whiteboard in my room I have a countdown till they come in December when I leave for good!

Link

I love my family!

1/13/06

Think and Ink

Good to be home. Shopping today was very frustrating—found three gorgeous dresses for coming-home party. The one I liked the most was $600, so I didn't get it. Got a really pretty pink one, though!

Link

Really good to be home!

Writing in her journal, Lauren communicates with herself about the various things that she's interested in or concerned about. Whatever she writes about helps to keep her identified and connected with her journal, SMJ, and the process of self-monitoring, and therefore helps foster a healthy obsession. If, as some researchers suggest, the benefits of keeping a journal result from an overall reduction of stress levels, it may not only help foster a healthy obsession, it might also improve sleep patterns and regulation of hormones.

Healthy obsession is the ultimate goal of the Sierras Solution. We'd love everyone to get there eventually. But, like many complex problems, weight control is only solved when all the pieces come together. Just eating under 20 grams of fat per day without maintaining ten thousand steps per day won't do it, nor will perfect self-monitoring without staying under 20 grams of fat per day.

You and the rest of your family are incredibly important to your new weight controller's long-term success. In the following sections, you will learn how to maximize your support for your child during your mutual pursuit of the three Simple Changes. Should you face some more intense challenges with your child, we recommend some other avenues to pursue—such as limit-setting and external support structures—to get your son or daughter back on track. First, let's look at some very common areas of concern, high-risk situations that need some extra attention to ensure success. Preparing for these will make them much more manageable.

Helping Your Child Prevent Missteps

The path to long-term weight control is strewn with obstacles and hazards; on any given day, you might encounter ambivalence, frustration, fear, pizza, television, the Internet, stress, lapses, high-risk situations, nagging, or teasing. If your child's healthy obsession is still under construction, some high-risk situations can prove challenging. Let's consider a few perennial situations and review how you can help your weight controller to master them.

Festive Gatherings at Homes of Friends or Family

These high-risk situations tend to invoke a free-spirit, "just have a good time" attitude. Although these qualities are great fun, they do challenge the focus and consistency necessary for effective weight control. But by using effective strategies, you and your weight controller can manage these stressors very successfully.

Consider Thanksgiving, a holiday that most Americans consider a well-justified eating frenzy and probably the extreme example of this category of high-risk situations. Here's a fairly typical Thanksgiving meal.

Foods/Serving Size	Calories
Turkey (no skin, half white, half dark meat)—3 ounces	148
Mashed potatoes—1 cup	222
Gravy—½ cup	61

(continued)

Foods/Serving Size	Calories
Stuffing—½ cup	250
Candied sweet potato—1	144
Cranberry sauce—2 tablespoons	52
Fresh fruit salad—½ cup	62
Celery—1 stalk	5
Carrots—½ cup	15
Bread—1 roll	71
Butter—1 pat	35
Pumpkin pie—2 slices	600
Whipped cream— 1/4 cup	200
Coffee	0
Total	**1,865**

This meal more than doubles the calorie-conscious limit of 800 calories for the biggest meal of the day. But many of these menu items pose no major problems: white-meat turkey without the skin, potatoes, fresh fruit salad, celery, and carrots. It's the stuffing, gravy, butter, pumpkin-pie crust, and whipped cream that pile on the fat and calories. By selecting the low-fat components of the classic Thanksgiving dinner, you can have an excellent meal and a wonderful time.

The Christmas season poses even greater risks for weight controllers. Unlike Thanksgiving, Easter, and parties at friends' houses, Christmas festivities last well beyond one particular day. Many people attend pre-Christmas parties and mini-celebrations, and find themselves surrounded by sugary treats at schools, offices, and in many homes. Many families enjoy baking Christmas cookies and other holiday foods—all during a time of year when the weather can make staying active especially challenging.

Several tricks of the trade are used by successful LTWCs during the holidays. These strategies apply equally well to eating at a friend's house or attending a birthday party.

Plan ahead. When you plan ahead, you can predict and control your world. Think about the next birthday party you'll attend. Who's going to be there and what kind of food will be served? Call the host and get a preview of the menu. You and your weight controller can make a tentative list of what you'll eat, who you'll talk to, and how to stay focused.

Keep self-monitoring a high priority. As routines change, consistency of self-monitoring often decreases, which compounds the challenges. Also, when you're at other people's homes and at parties, your ability to identify cooking methods and ingredients is diminished. So take your best shot and consult with your LTWC about food items in this situation. Research even shows that this kind of preparation alone can limit the damage caused by these stressors. Try to come up with a bottom-line estimate of the number of fat grams consumed for every day, even if the accuracy may not be great. The focus required for such estimates keeps weight controllers connected to their long-term goals and nurtures the healthy obsession.

We learned about how fat costs you nine calories per gram and has to be monitored very closely. It's as if you have twenty dollars to spend every day; you're going to watch where each "dollar" goes. This is like budgeting your money, but budgeting it on fat. That's how I think of spending my fat grams, like money.

—LAUREN S., FIFTEEN,
CALABASAS, CALIFORNIA
INITIAL WEIGHT LOSS:
FIFTY POUNDS IN FOUR MONTHS
SUSTAINED WEIGHT LOSS:
SIXTY-FOUR POUNDS FOR ONE YEAR

Avoid starvation before celebration. Starving before a big holiday meal can produce binge eating. Starving triggers a sense of deprivation and a very strong biological response to the sight of food. This biological response includes the secretion of insulin and saliva. In other words, if you eat nothing or very little before a big holiday meal or party, you will get incredibly hungry and are more likely to make bad decisions. A better approach is to enjoy low-fat, low-sugar foods for breakfast and lunch. Having a small snack just before leaving for the party may help as well.

Scope out the food scene. After arriving, you can quickly survey the available options. Perhaps there are fresh vegetables and other munchies that will work for you. You may also learn that the main course is a low-fat chicken, pasta, or fish dish. This knowledge may be the key to provide you with the control you need to keep away from the high-fat snacks.

Use a food plan. Once you are aware of what's available, you can develop a specific food plan for what you'll eat and a way of focusing on that plan. For example, you can hold a glass of diet soda or water and focus attention on the conversation instead of the food. You can also use this cue or some other cue (perhaps munching vegetables) to remind yourself of your immediate goals and your long-range goals. Try writing out this plan in advance and then seeing how your self-monitoring records match up immediately afterwards.

Refocus your holiday season. This suggestion goes well beyond an individual event or party. Holidays are traditionally centered on food and celebrations. You can break this tradition by paying attention to other people or special projects, and finding new, creative ways to relax. You might develop some skills in winter sports, such as ice skating or skiing, enjoy board games in front of a crackling fire, or read good books.

Feeling Bored, Anxious, Depressed, and Lazy

All four of these high-risk situations usually find your weight controller sitting around, trying to avoid unpleasant emotions, and looking for mindless distractions—a sure recipe for a lapse. One effective strategy used by many LTWCs is to use activity as a healthy coping skill. If your weight controller can learn to use activity to manage emotions and reduce sedentary activity more generally, the entire process gets a lot easier.

Move your body—it doesn't matter how long. Maintaining a high activity level helps weight controllers in many, many ways, including reducing appetite and improving mood. When you think of the billions of dollars spent on medications that curb appetite and improve mood, it's amazing to recognize that studies have shown that even ten minutes of brisk walking produces significant improvements in moods, for free!

Dr. Robert Thayer, a California State University psychologist, compared the results of eating a small candy bar (one-half ounce) versus taking a ten-

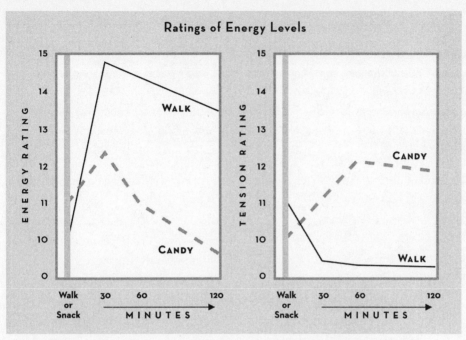

Ratings of Energy Levels

Based on Thayer, R. E. 1987. Energy, tiredness, and tension effects of a sugar snack versus moderate exercise. *Journal of Personality and Social Psychology* 52:119–125.

minute brisk walk. As shown in the figure above, walking led to more energy and lower tension, whereas the candy bar had the opposite effect.

Dr. Cheryl Hansen and her colleagues from Northern Arizona University wanted to see if ten, twenty, or thirty minutes of exercise produced different degrees of improvement in moods. The chart on page 186 shows what happened when their twenty-one college students rode exercise bikes at a fairly comfortable but somewhat strenuous intensity: 60 percent of maximum aerobic capacity. As you can see, even ten minutes on the bike produces substantial improvements in mood.

These improvements in mood send a message to your weight controller—keep reinforcing the ease and availability of this positive coping skill. We are firm believers in the statement *When the going gets rough, get going—even for just ten minutes*.

Talk to someone—anyone. When LTWCs are bored or depressed, they often rely on talking with friends, family members, and therapists to manage their moods. Such support can definitely reduce boredom, sadness, and other negative moods.

Encourage a Healthy
Obsession: Help
Your Child Follow the
Sierras Solution for Life

———

I guess the most disheartening thing is watching other people eating things that you can't eat. In the long run, I know I'm actually helping myself by the way I eat now. I had a totally different perspective after I came back from AOS. I just imagine that burger and fries or three slices of pizza sitting in my stomach. Do I want it? No. I also like chips and nachos, but when I think about clogging my arteries, I don't need it.

—LAUREN E., FIFTEEN,
HOUSTON, TEXAS
INITIAL WEIGHT LOSS:
FORTY-SIX POUNDS IN FOUR MONTHS
SUSTAINED WEIGHT LOSS:
FIFTY-TWO POUNDS FOR OVER ONE YEAR

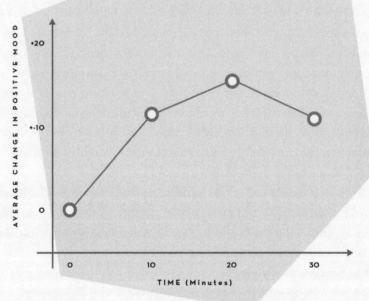

Impact of Duration of Exercise on Mood State

AVERAGE CHANGE IN POSITIVE MOOD

+20

+-10

0

TIME (Minutes)

0   10   20   30

Based on Hansen et al. "Exercise Duration and Mood State: How Much is Enough to Feel Better?" *Health Psychology,* 20 (2001):267–75.

Feeling Hungry and Having a Craving

Most diets focus on hunger and cravings as if they account for 98 percent of the problems of weight control. Yet, AOS students and alumni rank feelings of hunger and cravings relatively low among high-risk situations. Why is this? This program quiets hunger and cravings in many ways. Eating very low-fat, high-fiber, low-density foods decreases appetite, for example. Activity can also decrease hunger. But no one is immune to hunger or cravings, or mismanaging these feelings can derail them, at least temporarily. The next time your weight controller announces "I'm hungry" outside of regular mealtimes, consider discussing these questions:

- What do you think causes you to get hungry?
- Do you think that people around you or situations (like being in a certain restaurant or at a party) influence your hunger?

The research on hunger is clear: feeling hungry doesn't necessarily mean you physiologically require food. Many, many factors lurk behind the feeling of hunger.

Cravings are a very strong desire for food (perhaps stimulated by biological forces associated with weight loss or by not eating for a while) coupled with an idea. The idea could include a particular food or image of some food. The best antidotes for cravings are:

Distraction. Focus on other things, make a phone call.
Activity. Even a ten-minute walk, as noted earlier.
Eating. Something safe, particularly low-calorie-density foods.

I have amazing friends who are the most intellectual people I've ever met, and we talk. And sometimes, if I'm having a really bad day, I'll drive around with my best friend, Scott, for hours just talking. And we won't even be talking about what's wrong. We'll talk about what's wrong and then we'll talk about something random that leads back into what's wrong, and it just weaves in and out of that. And it helps so much.

—Josh S., fifteen,
Tucson, Arizona
Initial weight loss:
sixty-two pounds in five months
Sustained weight loss:
fifty-seven pounds for over one year

Encourage a Healthy Obsession: Help Your Child Follow the Sierras Solution for Life

---

A lapse is a silly little slipup that can happen and then you catch yourself. But when you relapse, you're just giving up. You're just saying, "Whatever. I'm done. I forfeit." Most people I know have had a lapse or two. I've had a lapse before and I was just, like, "You know what? You really can just do this." I know people who have had relapses, just given up, and they've gained a lot of their weight back.

—Vicki M., fourteen, Fairfax, Virginia
　Initial weight loss: sixty-six pounds in six months
　Sustained weight loss: fifty-four pounds for six additional months

What happens if you do give in to a high-risk situation? A person with a healthy obsession would fight like hell. At no time would you want a lapse to become a relapse.

Keep Lapses from Becoming Relapses

Our biology and our environment make it impossible for anyone to eat perfectly. A healthy obsession can help strengthen your weight controller's resolve, but you and your weight controller will do better if you accept the fact that you can't achieve perfection in eating. Lapses happen even to those who have a very healthy obsession. Lapses are inevitable—it's how you react to them that counts.

Understand that a lapse is not a tragedy. A lapse is a temporary problem, a temporary detour from the overall plan. A lapse does not have to lead to relapse, which is defined as a full-blown change back into old problematic patterns of eating and inactivity. LTWCs realize that eating an occasional high-fat ice-cream cone is a problem, not a catastrophe.

Use the resulting discomfort. Virtually all LTWCs feel some discomfort following a lapse, but the distinction between discomfort and tragedy is a key one for successful LTWCs. This disappointment or discomfort helps focus LTWCs on getting right back on track. Discomfort helps— guilt doesn't.

Are You *Really* Hungry?

The following factors influence the intensity of hunger. Ask yourself or your weight controller if one of these is responsible for a "hunger" attack.

Might Make You More Hungry

- Biology (fat cells)
- Seeing others around you eating, as at parties
- Consuming alcohol or using marijuana or other recreational drugs
- Feeling stressed, angry, frustrated, or bored
- Consuming fats
- Having negative thoughts ("I've blown it already today.")
- Being around foods, particularly highly appealing and attractive foods, as at a bakery, cookie store, or fast-food restaurant
- Stimuli that you associate with eating (riding in the car, watching TV)
- Consuming sugar by itself (as a snack), which can increase hunger within an hour or two
- Talking or thinking about food in great detail
- Time of day (when eating becomes strongly associated with certain times of day)
- Feeling tired
- Variety in your diet (more variety makes food more appealing)

Might Make You Less Hungry

- Positive emotions
- Fiber—consuming more can help you manage hunger
- Protein—consuming more can help you manage hunger
- Volume of food (high volumes of low-density foods)
- Activities—quick bouts of exercise can diminish cravings
- Eating lots of the same foods (blandness in the diet)
- Eating very low-fat foods

View it as a problem to be solved. If your child goes to a friend's house and eats some high-fat potato chips and regular soda, no one has died, a catastrophe hasn't occurred. The deviation from the plan simply warrants closer scrutiny. She'll look up the fat grams and calories and monitor what she ate. Then she'll consider alternatives that might have prevented the problem. For example, she'd realize that if she had brought her own baked chips and Diet Coke to her friend's house, she would have been just fine.

Guilt is the enemy, not the lapse itself. The only way lapses can become relapses is if the lapse is allowed to result in guilt or depression that overwhelms the LTWC's desire to succeed. So if your child eats four slices of pizza, he might feel bad about it, but he should consider it a problem to be solved and get right back on track. If he considers it a disaster, he may give up monitoring for the next week or month. This is what needs to be avoided at all costs.

Try making a deal with your weight controller. Both of you can agree that you will lapse occasionally and accept that you will not do the Sierras Solution perfectly. You can help each other when these inevitable lapses occur. You can also agree to redouble your efforts after a lapse to prevent the possibility of a relapse.

Make a sign for your house that says LAPSE ≠ RELAPSE. You can also rephrase the the following ideas and techniques and add them to the sign:

- Lapses are inevitable.
- No one does the Sierras Solution perfectly.
- Reexamine the situation that led to the lapse. What else could you have done to prevent the lapse from occurring?
- Go back to the fundamentals aggressively after a lapse: Eat very little fat for the next several days; get more than ten thousand steps every day; self-monitor everything.
- Revisit your Decision Balance Sheet—maybe redo it and hang it up on a closet door.
- Remind yourself of how much you've invested in your program and all of the benefits you've enjoyed.

There's no question that emotions can dramatically affect weight control. Managing stressors well can go a long way to ensuring that your child will become an LTWC. But sometimes it is not internal reactions but external distractions that can interfere with your child's focus on the plan. When that happens, setting appropriate limits can help your child succeed until he can once again be motivated by his own success.

Set Appropriate Limits

If your child is like most kids today, he loves to spend hours online, at MySpace, or playing video games. While every household has its own rules, we believe that if your child is consistently following the three Simple Changes, as well as living up to expectations at school and elsewhere, he should be allowed to continue to enjoy these activities without limits. But when these privileges appear to be getting in the way of staying on the Sierras Solution plan, it's time to limit them.

Use a behavior contract. If excessive time online is interfering with the plan, consider using a written behavioral contract similar to the reward-oriented contract. In addition to the eating, exercise, and self-monitoring goals, include one that limits time online. For example, "Goal #1: No more than two hours of screen time a day." If the goal is not met, instead of giving a reward, you create a consequence, such as limiting allowance or granting fewer privileges on weekends and evenings.

Negotiate the limits. Establishing these limits gets easier if you are able to negotiate them with your young weight controller. For example, you may have a number in mind, like two hours of screen time per day, but your weight controller currently averages six hours per day. You could suggest the limit of two hours, but have in mind a willingness to negotiate up to three or even four hours in the early stages. You'll be treating your young weight controller in a more adult fashion and this will produce greater cooperation.

At least four areas that have direct impact on weight control are worthy of consideration for setting limits.

Limit screen time. Surveys have indicated that children between the ages of two and seventeen with access to home computers and video games spend an average of five hours per day in front of a screen. In contrast, parents reported that children without computers or video games spent less than four hours per day in front of a screen.

As you might expect, screen time, a remarkably sedentary activity, is strongly correlated with weight problems in children and adolescents. Similarly, studies show that reducing screen time by setting limits can significantly reduce excess weight.

The American Academy of Pediatrics suggests that parents consider taking the following steps to control the screen time of their children:

- Watch only specific programs; do not turn the television on and let it run.
- Remove televisions and computers from bedrooms.
- Limit screen time viewing to two hours or less daily.
- Do not watch television or computer screens during meals.
- Watch shows with children and discuss what is shown.
- Substitute reading or playtime for television or screen time.
- Teach children the difference between advertisements and program content.

Eliminate high-fat foods in the home. Presuming your LTWC is already on the plan, this limit is a reminder for other family members. If you have an older, argumentative teenager who doesn't accept this, ask her to consider what would happen if one of the adults were a recovering alcoholic. Would the other adults in the household drink alcohol with dinner in that case? The same approach applies to weight controllers.

You'll want to make it clear to every household member that high-fat foods are contraband in your home. If they emerge, for whatever reason, you will toss them out as soon as you find them.

When you present this limit, emphasize that this alternative style of eating will improve the health of everyone in the family. Say, "As your parent, one of my major jobs is to protect your health. Eating this way will do that. We're also going to have a lot of fun with it and make sure the food tastes great. After a while, you won't miss the higher-fat foods at all."

Limit drinks with calories. Remember, the vast majority of Americans drink hundreds of calories per day in the form of fruit juices, specialty coffee drinks, and other liquids. Studies show that drinking high-calorie beverages actually can increase appetite and result in consuming hundreds, sometimes even thousands, of extra calories per day that do you no good and that do not reduce hunger. For this reason, the American Academy of Pediatrics recommends drinking diet soft drinks instead of regular (high-sugar) soft drinks.

Explaining the Danger of High-Fat Food to the Family

One way of making the danger of high-fat food clear, even to very young children, is to use their fingers for a demonstration. Ask them to feel the pad of the fingertip of the middle finger of the left hand. Ask them to flick that finger with their other hand and notice how soft it is. Then ask them to turn over their left hand and flick their middle finger's fingernail. They'll notice the hardness and they can actually hear the clicking sound upon flicking that finger. Tell them that their arteries, the main blood vessels in their bodies that carry nutrients to all of their cells, are supposed to feel like the soft part of their fingers. When people eat too much fat their arteries become like fingernails instead of the soft parts of fingers. This is what causes most heart attacks.

The Sierras Solution rule on beverages is simple: Eat your calories. Don't drink them, except for skim milk. It's a simple rule that every child can understand.

Should these limits not produce noticeable changes, you might consider supplementing your efforts with some outside structure.

Provide Structure

Once your weight controller has consistently followed the three simple changes in the Sierras Solution for six to twelve weeks, now's the time to think about whether he has made good progress. How much weight has he lost? Assuming he had at least twenty pounds to lose, you could expect weight loss of a least half a pound per week (assuming no additional growth) after twelve weeks of consistent adherence to the Sierras Solution. He gets credit for a three-pound weight loss for each half-inch increase in height. So, if his weight stayed at 180 pounds even though he grew half an inch, consider that the same as losing three pounds.

If this hasn't happened, or if your weight controller isn't satisfied with his progress, or if you have not been able to nudge him out of the shock and ambivalence stage, despite numerous attempts, the next step is to consider adding structure to help accelerate change and foster development of a healthy obsession. Adding structure can range from introducing simple changes to substantial and potentially more powerful interventions. As with the process of adding the Simple Changes, you can keep adding these interventions until the goal is achieved.

GET A LITTLE HELP FROM YOUR FRIENDS

Involve a friend of your child's who is also overweight. If your weight controller has a friend also following the Sierras Solution, they can participate in activities together like walking in the morning before school, participating in new sports, or even sharing a personal trainer. The personal trainer comes to one house, both weight controllers participate, and the families split the cost. You can also arrange Sierras-friendly dinners together.

JOIN A SELF-HELP GROUP

This an excellent way to add structure and keep your weight controller focused on the goal. There are two well-known and widely available self-help groups in the United States and Canada.

Take Off Pounds Sensibly (TOPS). Founded in 1948, TOPS has two hundred thousand members and ten thousand chapters operating in the United States, Canada, and several other countries. To find the group meeting nearest you, go to www.tops.org, click on "Meetings," and enter your zip code. The authors did this and found twenty-five, seven, and five chapters, respectively, within ten miles of each of our homes. Each chapter lists its meeting address and time, as well as the name of chapter leaders with phone numbers. Many chapters welcome teenagers, and many AOS and Wellspring alumni have benefited from attending TOPS meetings to stay on program.

TOPS focuses on self-monitoring, healthful eating, and staying active in a fashion consistent with the principles of the Sierras Solution. While

TOPS doesn't advocate a very low-fat approach or the use of pedometers and the ten-thousand-step goal, it can still be very useful to keep your weight controller focused and motivated. The cost is also low. You will need to become a member (which currently costs $24 in the U.S., $30 in Canada) and may need to pay nominal chapter fees. Each chapter sets its own fees to cover operating expenses.

These benefits outweigh the drawbacks of TOPS, which include the fact that some TOPS groups include people with substantial problems who can distract from the focus on the behaviors required for successful long-term weight control. TOPS group leaders also have minimal training.

If you can't find an appropriate chapter nearby, TOPS offers starter kits that your weight controller could use to start a chapter at his high school. Costs are minimal.

Weight Watchers. The only other nonprofessional approach that follows enough of the science of weight loss to warrant recommendation is Weight Watchers. Weight Watchers also encourages healthful eating and self-monitoring.

There are over twenty thousand Weight Watchers groups around the country. To find a meeting, go to www.weightwatchers.com and click on "Find a Meeting." The authors did this and found thirty-three, eleven, and three chapters, respectively, within ten miles of each of our homes.

Prior to March 2003, Weight Watchers had permitted children and teens to participate in its adult programs. Then Weight Watchers adopted a new policy refusing all children below age ten and only accepting ages ten through sixteen with a doctor's referral. So you will need a note from your doctor to gain entry for your weight controller if she is sixteen or under.

Although Weight Watchers is famous for its Points program, Weight Watchers also offers a Core program that doesn't use points but rather focuses on self-monitoring, education, and support. While popular, the Weight Watchers Points program fails the simplicity test. It assigns points to every food based on a complex formula primarily factoring in fat and fiber content. To use it, participants must look up the value for everything they eat, something particularly challenging in parties and restaurants, in our view. In contrast, a ten-year-old with just a little training can read a label and determine how much fat each food contains. The simple principles for ordering very low-fat food that we've presented and illustrated can help you and your weight controller negotiate almost any situation outside of the home. We also view high-fiber foods as helpful, and have noted several other ancillary guidelines, but the primary emphasis remains very simple, easily adapted to any situation, and sustainable.

Weight controllers who attend Weight Watchers meetings can remember that they won't benefit much from buying Weight Watchers products at these meetings. Just follow the Core program and use the weekly meetings as an opportunity to improve your focus and commitment. Costs amount to about ten to fifteen dollars per week. As with TOPS, the trainers receive minimal training and certainly are not professional therapists. Also, some members can prove distracting.

Other approaches. The other nonprofessional approaches, like Overeaters Anonymous and Jenny Craig, have numerous flaws in their approaches from a scientific perspective. We don't recommend any other nonprofessional approach aside from TOPS and Weight Watchers for this reason.

Get Help from a Professional

Many hospitals and medical centers offer professional weight management programs that can help more kids with greater success than the nonprofessional programs listed above.

Look for programs directed by psychologists or other mental-health professionals with expertise in cognitive-behavior therapy, the approach that has the best track record by far and forms the basis of much of the Sierras Solution. The better weight management programs are open-ended, providing help for unlimited periods of time and definitely not less than one year. Longer-term programs tend to produce better outcomes.

Many psychologists and therapists operate weight-management programs as a component of their practice. For some, it's their main focus. The following three organizations also have listings of mental-health professionals in virtually every area of the United States:

1. Association for Advancement of Behavioral and Cognitive Therapies. Go to www.abct.org and click on "Find a therapist."
2. American Psychological Association. Go to www.apa.org and click on "Find a psychologist."
3. National Association of Social Workers. Go to www.helpstarts here.org and click on "Find a social worker."

Calls to local hospitals and to the psychology departments of local colleges and universities may prove helpful.

As we go to press, our organization is planning to launch an after-school version of our programs in select markets. Called Wellspring Community Programs, these after-school programs should be available in one or two cities by the end of 2007. Please visit www.wellspringprograms.com for more information.

IMMERSION PROGRAMS

Programs like AOS and our Wellspring Camps immerse weight controllers in a very structured world of healthy living and provide them with education, encouragement, and cognitive-behavior therapy to help them change. This intensive experience typically results in rapid weight loss and builds tremendous momentum to help students and campers develop a healthy obsession. They can see that they really can succeed, perhaps for the first time.

It's unfortunate that it is so challenging to compete with the biological and environmental factors that make it hard to lose weight. So it's certainly possible that you may not be able to overcome these barriers even with help from professionals dedicated to the same scientific principles as the Sierras Solution. If this is the case, a scientifically based immersion program can make a huge difference.

If you're considering an alternative immersion program such as a traditional diet or weight-loss camp, consider asking the questions in the box titled "Ten Questions to Ask if You Are Considering a Weight-Loss Camp" (see next page) before spending thousands of dollars on an approach that is unlikely to be successful in helping your child achieve his or her goal.

A Last Word

AOS's motto, *mens et salvere*, is a Latin phrase meaning "mind and health." Or, as we explain to new students, "The development of the mind progresses in lockstep with overall health."

Weight control is a two-way street. On one side, improvements in health

Ten Questions to Ask if You Are Considering a Weight-Loss Camp

1. What was last year's average weekly weight loss at camp?
2. What are the camp's long-term results? What percentage of campers maintain or continue weight loss at home?
3. Who designed the weight-loss program? What are their credentials? Is the program design scientifically based?
4. Is counseling (particularly cognitive-behavior therapy) offered by qualified therapists?
5. If so, do the therapists work full-time at the camp during the summer? Does each camper have an individual therapist assigned to her? Do therapists continue to work with campers after campers return home?
6. How are families involved?
7. How many campers return each year? Did they regain weight? Will new campers feel left out because of cliques from prior years?
8. How large is the camp? Is it a manageable size where the camp director knows each and every camper?
9. Can we talk to several families of campers who have maintained or continued weight loss from last summer?
10. Does the camp demonstrate improvements in self-esteem and overall well-being?

via long-term weight control do wonders for emotions, mood, energy, outlook, and academic performance. Health improves the mind.

On the other side, you now understand that the path to health via long-term weight control requires ample and frequent use of the mind. As we often say at AOS, it's "mind over taco." Every single aspect of the Sierras Solution—the three Simple Changes, a healthy obsession, strategies to escape frustration and avoid and mitigate lapses—requires thought and focus. This isn't always easy for children and teens. But in time, it can be done with your love and support.

Mens et salvere. Our mind and body are connected—not in some pseudoscientific kind of way, but in several very specific ways, substantiated by our experience with thousands of young weight controllers, and backed up by decades of scientific research.

When we established Academy of the Sierras, our goal was, and remains, to help as many children as possible. Several years in, we are very proud to be part of a revolutionary approach that one day might make the difference for millions of kids and their families.

We hope that you're able to use the Sierras Solution as a tool to help your child become a long-term weight controller. You've taken a giant first step by reading this book. We applaud you for making such a huge commitment to your child's health and future, and your own. *Mens et salvere.*

PART 4

The Sierras Solution Eating Plan

Chapter 11

The Sierras Solution Menu Plan: Six Weeks of Delicious, Satisfying, Nutritious Meals for Your Family

You won't have to work that hard to convince your family to adopt the Sierras Solution program once they've tasted these meals. Every one of the menus and recipes in our program was created by our Culinary Institute of America–trained chef, culinary instructor Erin Gaughan, in consultation with other registered dieticians and nutritionists, and is the reflection of years of research, creativity, and on-site fine-tuning.

Each day on the program, you and your weight controller will eat the same very low-fat, low-calorie-density, high-protein, high-fiber menu enjoyed by the students at AOS. You'll savor three delicious meals and two healthy snacks of what we call "controlled food"—meals with specific portions recommended (which are listed in each day of the meal plan). But you can also eat an *unlimited amount* of low-calorie-density "uncontrolled" foods, such as soups, fresh fruit, and salad, as well as nonfat, high-protein items such as various fat-free yogurts, fat-free tuna salad, fat-free egg salad, and fat-free cottage cheese. These uncontrolled foods provide weight controllers the opportunity and latitude to make their own food choices.

A typical day of controlled foods includes 1,200 calories, 10 grams of fat, 50 grams of protein, and 30 grams of fiber. Uncontrolled foods will add to these totals—often significantly, particularly at first, or when your weight controller might experience some frustration. But remember: On the Sierras Solution program, there is no caloric goal. If you or your weight controller is hungry, you both can have as much uncontrolled food as you like until you are satisfied. All we ask is that you and your weight controller remember Simple Change #1 (limit total fat to less than 20 grams) and Simple Change #3 (record what you eat—self-monitor—so you'll have an opportunity to reflect on your intake on a daily and weekly basis, and note any trends, positive or negative).

We've found that very few weight controllers have any difficulty adopting this eating plan. In making these recipes very low in fat, we've changed the nutrition profile of familiar foods, but we've worked hard not to change the tastes. In the meal plan, you'll be introduced to foods that have the same flavor and feel as the foods you both are used to, but that also meet the Sierras Solution's nutrition parameters. That's part of what makes this program so successful— we help weight controllers to change their lifestyle permanently because the food on the program is as appealing as the food they're used to eating!

Before you start the plan, take a look at the Week One Shopping List on page 301. Better yet, bring this book to the grocery store. Each week has a corresponding shopping list, for your convenience.

We encourage you to follow the plan as closely as you can for the first six weeks. Doing so will help you get the feel for cooking the Sierras Solutions way and will teach you all of our secret techniques for preserving flavor while ditching fat. Always focus on the pleasure of the process: shop together, prepare the meals together, and enjoy some relaxed bonding time. Your overarching goal is to turn these six weeks of meal plans into a natural, delicious, healthy way of life for your weight controller—and yourself. Bon appetit!

Sierra Solution Staple Meals

On the days when you or your weight controller just can't follow the meal plan—whether you have a late night at work, or your weight controller has no time to prepare lunch for school—substitute these staple meals, and you'll stay right on track.

The
Sierras
Solution
Eating
Plan
—
204

BREAKFAST—SELECT ONE	CALORIES	FAT GRAMS
1 serving Special K (with fat-free milk)	200	0
1 serving Cheerios (with fat-free milk)	165	0
1 serving Corn Flakes (with fat-free milk)	165	0
1 serving Raisin Bran (with fat-free milk)	280	0
1 serving Shredded Wheat (with fat-free milk)	210	0
1 serving fat-free yogurt with banana	230	0

LUNCH OR DINNER

BREAD—SELECT ONE	CALORIES	FAT GRAMS
1 pita bread	90	0
1 fat-free flour tortilla	90	0
2 pieces fat-free, whole-wheat bread	70	0
1 hot dog bun	110	1.5

CONTENTS—SELECT ONE	CALORIES	FAT GRAMS
3 ounces tuna fish, canned in water	110	2.5
3 ounces fat-free turkey breast	90	0
1 fat-free Ball Park regular hot dog	40	0
1 fat-free Ball Park beef hot dog	45	0
1 Ball Park turkey frank	45	0
2 ounces (6 slices) Hillshire Deli Select pastrami	60	1
2 ounces Healthy Choice roast beef	60	1.5
½ cup Egg Beaters (2 egg whites)	60	0
2 ounces fat-free cheddar cheese	82	0
2 ounces fat-free American cheese	82	0
2 ounces fat-free mozzarella	84	0
2 tablespoons Peanut Wonder	100	2.5
1 tablespoon jam, jelly, or preserves	65	0

CONDIMENTS—SELECT AS MANY AS YOU LIKE	CALORIES	FAT GRAMS
1 tablespoon fat-free mayonnaise	10	0
1 tablespoon yellow mustard	15	0
1 tablespoon ketchup	15	0
1 tablespoon honey mustard	15	0
1 teaspoon horseradish	2	0
1 large dill pickle	12	0

The Sierras Solution
Menu Plan: Six Weeks
of Delicious, Satisfying,
Nutritious Meals for
Your Family

———

CONDIMENTS—SELECT AS MANY AS YOU LIKE	CALORIES	FAT GRAMS
1 tablespoon sweet pickle relish	20	0
1 cup shredded/chopped lettuce	7	0
1 cup fresh spinach	7	0
1 thin slice onion	4	0
1 thick slice tomato	5	0
½ red bell pepper	14	0
1 ounce sliced cucumber	4	0
4 carrot sticks (1½ ounces)	18	0

DELICIOUS ADD-ONS TO ANY LUNCH OR DINNER

One of the things weight controllers love about the Sierras Solution meal plan is how much variety it offers. Below you'll find a list of dozens of appetizers, dips, sauces, side dishes, soups, and salads. You and your weight controller can choose *any* one that you like and add it to *any* lunch or dinner. Mix and match to your heart's content—just remember to add the fat grams to your journal. See Appetizers, Dips, and Sauces (page 227) and Side Dishes, Soups, and Salads (page 286).

ADD-ONS FOR EVERY LUNCH AND DINNER	CALORIES	FAT GRAMS
All Choked Up Artichoke Dip	74.8	1
All Curried Up Dip/Spread	63	0
All Steamed Up Artichokes	78	0
Asparagus with Dip	50	0
Baked Light French Fries	175	0
Baked Potato Latkes	188	0
Barbecue Sauce	21.8	0.2
Blue-Stuffed Tomatoes	120	2
Bruschetta, Anyone?	178	1.4
Candied Carrots	124	2
Cheesy Broccoli Bake	92	0
Creamy Mushroom Soup	142	0.5
Crispy Panko Shrimp Appetizers	106	1.5
Curried Cauliflower Bake	74	1
Easiest Rice Pilaf Ever	63.3	0
Fine Herb Sauce	49.5	0.3

The
Sierras
Solution
Eating
Plan
—
206

Add-ons for Every Lunch and Dinner	Calories	Fat Grams
Fall Fruit w/Vanilla-Maple Dip	79	0
Green Bean Casserole	65	0
Guiltless Mac and Cheese	260	1
Herb-Roasted Vegetables	55	1
Italian Vegetable Salad	27.8	1.2
Joe's Wild, Wild Mushroom Risotto	210	2
Leek and Gold Potato Soup	141	0
Mexican Spring Rolls	45	1
No Crying Onion Quesadillas	109.5	3.2
No-Fry Sweet Potato French Fries	74	1
Roasted Candied Acorn Squash	49.2	0
Roasted Caramelized Onions	74	0
Roasted Garlic Hummus	39	0.3
Smoked Turkey and Cilantro Spread	115	1.5
South of the Border Dip	20.5	0.3
Southwestern Cheese Dip	65.5	0
Spinach Dip	59.8	0.5
Spinach, Raspberry, and Mandarin Orange Salad	62.5	1
Sweet and Sour Coleslaw	44.8	0.2
Sweet and Spicy Turkey Pinwheels	42	1
Sweet and Tart Carrots and Apples	137	1.5
Sweet Potato Kugel	103	0.5
Wild Mushroom Crostini	74	0
Zucchini Fingers	119	1.5

Recommended Low-Fat and Fat-Free Snacks

You and your weight controller need never lack for something to snack on. Here are a few popular options that fit right in line with Simple Change #1.

Low- and Fat-Free Snacks	Portion Size	Calories	Fat Grams
Air-popped popcorn	1 cup	40	0
Apple Cinnamon Quaker rice cakes	1 package – 0.5 ounces	50	0
Beef jerky	1 package – 0.9 ounces	70	1

Low- and Fat-Free Snacks	Portion Size	Calories	Fat Grams
Caramel Corn Quaker rice cakes	1 package – 0.5 ounces	50	0
Fat-free muffins	1.65 ounces	130	0
Fat-free pretzels	1¼-ounce package	120	0
Fig Newman's	2 cookies	120	0
Fruit (most varieties)	1 piece	70	0
No Pudge brownies	¹⁄₁₂ package, prepared	90	0
Raisins	1½-ounce box	130	0

The
Sierras
Solution
Eating
Plan

——

208

Week One

		CALORIES	FAT GRAMS
Monday	**Breakfast**		
	Sierra Blueberry Pancakes	76	0.25
	Lunch		
	Tuna Patties	265	1.25
	Optional side dish/appetizer		
	Snack		
	Dinner		
	Southwestern Chicken Rollatini	224	2
	Optional side dish/appetizer		
	Snack		
	Total Calorie and Fat Intake from Main Courses:	**565**	**3.5**
Tuesday	**Breakfast**		
	The Popeye Special Omelet	110	0.5
	Lunch		
	Crispy Chicken Fingers	220	1.5
	Optional side dish/appetizer		
	Snack		
	Dinner		
	Roasted Salmon Fillet	166	5.5
	Optional side dish/appetizer		
	Snack		
	Total Calorie and Fat Intake from Main Courses:	**496**	**7.5**
Wednesday	**Breakfast**		
	AOS Breakfast Stacker	89.5	2.1
	Lunch		
	Kickin' Chicken Wrap	302	2
	Optional side dish/appetizer		
	Snack		

The Sierras Solution
Menu Plan: Six Weeks
of Delicious, Satisfying,
Nutritious Meals for
Your Family

—

		Calories	Fat Grams
Wednesday	**Dinner**		
	Parmesan-Encrusted Tilapia	235	4
	Optional side dish/appetizer		
	Snack		
	Total Calorie and Fat Intake from Main Courses:	**425.6**	**7.5**
Thursday	**Breakfast**		
	Sorry, Charlie, Breakfast Melt	265	3
	Lunch		
	Mandarin Chicken Wraps	240	2
	Optional side dish/appetizer		
	Snack		
	Dinner		
	No Bones About It Garlic Chicken	142	3
	Optional side dish/appetizer		
	Snack		
	Total Calorie and Fat Intake from Main Courses:	**562**	**7.5**
Friday	**Breakfast**		
	Emu Scramble	263	1
	Lunch		
	Cheesy Chicken and Mushroom Casserole	240	1.5
	Optional side dish/appetizer		
	Snack		
	Dinner		
	Fresno Beef Stir-Fry	226	5
	Optional side dish/appetizer		
	Snack		
	Total Calorie and Fat Intake from Main Courses:	**729**	**7.5**
Saturday	**Breakfast**		
	Huevos Rancheros Burritos	172	0
	Lunch		
	Hakuna Matata Frittata	147	1.5
	Optional side dish/appetizer		

The
Sierras
Solution
Eating
Plan
——
210

		CALORIES	FAT GRAMS
Saturday	**Snack**		
	Dinner		
	Five-Alarm Roasted Chicken	158	3
	Optional side dish/appetizer		
	Snack		
	Total Calorie and Fat Intake from Main Courses:	477	4.5
Sunday	**Breakfast**		
	Zenaida's Quiche	202	0
	Lunch		
	Who Are You Calling Chicken? Enchiladas	152	1.5
	Optional side dish/appetizer		
	Snack		
	Dinner		
	All Gobbled Up Roasted Turkey	151	1
	Optional side dish/appetizer		
	Snack		
	Total Calorie and Fat Intake from Main Courses:	505	2.5

The Sierras Solution
Menu Plan: Six Weeks
of Delicious, Satisfying,
Nutritious Meals for
Your Family

———

Week Two

		CALORIES	FAT GRAMS
Monday	**Breakfast**		
	All Wrapped Up	177	1
	Lunch		
	Apricot Ginger Pita	190.1	1.3
	Optional side dish/appetizer		
	Snack		
	Dinner		
	Heavenly Basil Pasta	238	2
	Optional side dish/appetizer		
	Snack		
	Total Calorie and Fat Intake from Main Courses:	**605.1**	**4.3**
Tuesday	**Breakfast**		
	AOS Taters and Eggs	158	0.1
	Lunch		
	Sweet and Sour Lychee Chicken Stir-Fry	172.5	1.7
	Optional side dish/appetizer		
	Snack		
	Dinner		
	Chicken Piccata	130	1.5
	Optional side dish/appetizer		
	Snack		
	Total Calorie and Fat Intake from Main Courses:	**460.5**	**3.3**
Wednesday	**Breakfast**		
	Oh, My, Oatmeal Bake	103	0.8
	Lunch		
	Sharon's Chicken Taco Salad	306	3.7
	Optional side dish/appetizer		
	Snack		

The
Sierras
Solution
Eating
Plan
———
212

		CALORIES	FAT GRAMS
Wednesday	**Dinner**		
	Apple of My Eye Pork Stir-Fry	351	3
	Optional side dish/appetizer		
	Snack		
	Total Calorie and Fat Intake from Main Courses:	**760**	**7.5**
Thursday	**Breakfast**		
	Candy Apple Breakfast Pudding	208	1.5
	Lunch		
	Not Your Grandma's Chicken Salad Pita	189	2.6
	Optional side dish/appetizer		
	Snack		
	Dinner		
	Chicken Marsala	198	1.5
	Optional side dish/appetizer		
	Snack		
	Total Calorie and Fat Intake from Main Courses:	**595**	**5.6**
Friday	**Breakfast**		
	Sierra Blueberry Pancakes	76	0.25
	Lunch		
	Quiche Florentine	111	2
	Optional side dish/appetizer		
	Snack		
	Dinner		
	Balsamic Baked Chicken	173	1.5
	Optional side dish/appetizer		
	Snack		
	Total Calorie and Fat Intake from Main Courses:	**360**	**3.75**
Saturday	**Breakfast**		
	Sorry, Charlie, Breakfast Melt	265	3
	Lunch		
	Crabby Portobellos	148	0
	Optional side dish/appetizer		

The Sierras Solution
Menu Plan: Six Weeks
of Delicious, Satisfying,
Nutritious Meals for
Your Family

———

213

		CALORIES	FAT GRAMS
Saturday	**Snack**		
	Dinner		
	Cheesy Chicken and Mushroom Casserole	240	1.5
	Optional side dish/appetizer		
	Snack		
	Total Calorie and Fat Intake from Main Courses:	**653**	**4.5**
Sunday	**Breakfast**		
	AOS Breakfast Stacker	89.5	2.1
	Lunch		
	Sweet Potato Couscous	238	2
	Optional side dish/appetizer		
	Snack		
	Dinner		
	Orange You Glad It's Scallops?	154	2
	Optional side dish/appetizer		
	Snack		
	Total Calorie and Fat Intake from Main Courses:	**481.5**	**6.1**

The
Sierras
Solution
Eating
Plan

—

214

Week Three

		CALORIES	FAT GRAMS
Monday	**Breakfast**		
	Mama Mia's Breakfast Calzone	110	0.5
	Lunch		
	Quiche Florentine	111	2
	Optional side dish/appetizer		
	Snack		
	Dinner		
	Very Veggie Stuffed Bell Pepper	165	0
	Optional side dish/appetizer		
	Snack		
	Total Calorie and Fat Intake from Main Courses:	**386**	**2.5**
Tuesday	**Breakfast**		
	Sorry, Charlie, Breakfast Melt	265	3
	Lunch		
	Sharon's Chicken Taco Salad	306	3.7
	Optional side dish/appetizer		
	Snack		
	Dinner		
	Acorn Squash Ravioli	315	2
	Optional side dish/appetizer		
	Snack		
	Total Calorie and Fat Intake from Main Courses:	**886**	**8.7**
Wednesday	**Breakfast**		
	The Popeye Special Omelet	110	0.5
	Lunch		
	Sweet Potato Couscous	204	1
	Optional side dish/appetizer		
	Snack		

The Sierras Solution
Menu Plan: Six Weeks
of Delicious, Satisfying,
Nutritious Meals for
Your Family

———

			CALORIES	FAT GRAMS
Wednesday	**Dinner** Mango-licious Barbecue Shrimp Optional side dish/appetizer		390	5
	Snack			
	Total Calorie and Fat Intake from Main Courses:		**704**	**6.5**
Thursday	**Breakfast** Sierra Blueberry Pancakes		76	0.25
	Lunch Reedley's Best Pizza Optional side dish/appetizer		238	3
	Snack			
	Dinner My Big Fat Greek Chicken Optional side dish/appetizer		159	2
	Snack			
	Total Calorie and Fat Intake from Main Courses:		**473**	**5.25**
Friday	**Breakfast** Emu Scramble		146	2
	Lunch Happy as a Clam Pasta Optional side dish/appetizer		301	3
	Snack			
	Dinner Home on the Range Buffaloaf Optional side dish/appetizer		254	4
	Snack			
	Total Calorie and Fat Intake from Main Courses:		**701**	**9**
Saturday	**Breakfast** AOS Breakfast Stacker		89.5	2.1
	Lunch Crispy Chicken Fingers Optional side dish/appetizer		176	1.5

The
Sierras
Solution
Eating
Plan
———
216

		CALORIES	FAT GRAMS
Saturday	**Snack**		
	Dinner		
	Spaghetti Bison Pie	420	3
	Optional side dish/appetizer		
	Snack		
	Total Calorie and Fat Intake from Main Courses:	685.5	6.6
Sunday	**Breakfast**		
	Quiche Florentine	111	2
	Lunch		
	Hakuna Matata Frittata	147	1.5
	Optional side dish/appetizer		
	Snack		
	Dinner		
	Eat Your Spinach Manicotti	325	0.5
	Optional side dish/appetizer		
	Snack		
	Total Calorie and Fat Intake from Main Courses:	583	4

The Sierras Solution
Menu Plan: Six Weeks
of Delicious, Satisfying,
Nutritious Meals for
Your Family

———

Week Four

		Calories	Fat Grams
Monday	**Breakfast**		
	AOS Taters and Eggs	158	0.1
	Lunch		
	Crabby Portobellos	148	0
	Optional side dish/appetizer		
	Snack		
	Dinner		
	Balsamic Baked Chicken	173	1.5
	Optional side dish/appetizer		
	Snack		
	Total Calorie and Fat Intake from Main Courses:	**479**	**1.6**
Tuesday	**Breakfast**		
	Oh, My, Oatmeal	103	0.8
	Lunch		
	Not Your Grandma's Chicken Salad Pita	189	2.6
	Optional side dish/appetizer		
	Snack		
	Dinner		
	All Juiced Up Pork Tenderloin	221	5
	Optional side dish/appetizer		
	Snack		
	Total Calorie and Fat Intake from Main Courses:	**513**	**8.4**
Wednesday	**Breakfast**		
	Candy Apple Breakfast Pudding	208	1.5
	Lunch		
	Southwestern Chicken Rollatini	224	2
	Optional side dish/appetizer		
	Snack		

The
Sierras
Solution
Eating
Plan
—
218

		CALORIES	FAT GRAMS
Wednesday	**Dinner**		
	Heavenly Basil Pasta	238	2
	Optional side dish/appetizer		
	Snack		
	Total Calorie and Fat Intake from Main Courses:	**670**	**5.5**
Thursday	**Breakfast**		
	Huevos Rancheros Burritos	172	0
	Lunch		
	All Gobbled Up Roasted Turkey Breast	151	1
	Optional side dish/appetizer		
	Snack		
	Dinner		
	Apple of My Eye Pork Stir-Fry	351	3
	Optional side dish/appetizer		
	Snack		
	Total Calorie and Fat Intake from Main Courses:	**674**	**4**
Friday	**Breakfast**		
	Zenaida's Quiche	202	0
	Lunch		
	Sharon's Chicken Taco Salad	306	3.7
	Optional side dish/appetizer		
	Snack		
	Dinner		
	Pasta with Garlic Shrimp and Olives	290	2.5
	Optional side dish/appetizer		
	Snack		
	Total Calorie and Fat Intake from Main Courses:	**798**	**6.2**
Saturday	**Breakfast**		
	All Wrapped Up	177	1
	Lunch		
	Who Are You Calling Chicken? Enchiladas	152	1.5
	Optional side dish/appetizer		

The Sierras Solution Menu Plan: Six Weeks of Delicious, Satisfying, Nutritious Meals for Your Family

—

219

		CALORIES	FAT GRAMS
Saturday	**Snack**		
	Dinner		
	Pork Chops au Poivre	167	4
	Optional side dish/appetizer		
	Snack		
	Total Calorie and Fat Intake from Main Courses:	**496**	**6.5**
Sunday	**Breakfast**		
	Mama Mia's Breakfast Calzone	110	0.5
	Lunch		
	Mandarin Chicken Wrap	155	1.5
	Optional side dish/appetizer		
	Snack		
	Dinner		
	Parmesan-Encrusted Tilapia	235	4
	Optional side dish/appetizer		
	Snack		
	Total Calorie and Fat Intake from Main Courses:	**500**	**6**

The
Sierras
Solution
Eating
Plan

—

220

Week Five

		CALORIES	FAT GRAMS
Monday	**Breakfast**		
	Emu Scramble	146	2
	Lunch		
	Sharon's Chicken Taco Salad	306	3.7
	Optional side dish/appetizer		
	Snack		
	Dinner		
	Acorn Squash Ravioli	315	2
	Optional side dish/appetizer		
	Snack		
	Total Calorie and Fat Intake from Main Courses:	**713.5**	**4.5**
Tuesday	**Breakfast**		
	The Popeye Special Omelet	110	0.5
	Lunch		
	Crispy Chicken Fingers	220	1.5
	Optional side dish/appetizer		
	Snack		
	Dinner		
	Roasted Salmon Fillet	166	5.5
	Optional side dish/appetizer		
	Snack		
	Total Calorie and Fat Intake from Main Courses:	**496**	**7.5**
Wednesday	**Breakfast**		
	AOS Breakfast Stacker	89.5	2.1
	Lunch		
	Kickin' Chicken Wrap	101.1	1.4
	Optional side dish/appetizer		
	Snack		

The Sierras Solution Menu Plan: Six Weeks of Delicious, Satisfying, Nutritious Meals for Your Family

———

		CALORIES	FAT GRAMS
Wednesday	**Dinner**		
	Eat Your Spinach Manicotti	325	0.5
	Optional side dish/appetizer		
	Snack		
	Total Calorie and Fat Intake from Main Courses:	**515.6**	**4**
Thursday	**Breakfast**		
	All Wrapped Up	265	3
	Lunch		
	Mandarin Chicken Wrap	155	1.5
	Optional side dish/appetizer		
	Snack		
	Dinner		
	No Bones About It Garlic Chicken	142	3
	Optional side dish/appetizer		
	Snack		
	Total Calorie and Fat Intake from Main Courses:	**562**	**7.5**
Friday	**Breakfast**		
	Oh, My, Oatmeal	263	1
	Lunch		
	Cheesy Chicken and Mushroom Casserole	240	1.5
	Optional side dish/appetizer		
	Snack		
	Dinner		
	Sharon's Chicken Taco Salad	306	3.7
	Optional side dish/appetizer		
	Snack		
	Total Calorie and Fat Intake from Main Courses:	**809**	**6.2**
Saturday	**Breakfast**		
	Quiche Florentine	111	2
	Lunch		
	Hakuna Matata Frittata	147	1.5
	Optional side dish/appetizer		

The
Sierras
Solution
Eating
Plan
—
222

		CALORIES	FAT GRAMS
Saturday	**Snack**		
	Dinner		
	Five-Alarm Roasted Chicken	224	2
	Optional side dish/appetizer		
	Snack		
	Total Calorie and Fat Intake from Main Courses:	**482**	**5.5**
Sunday	**Breakfast**		
	Sierra Blueberry Pancakes	76	0.25
	Lunch		
	Who Are You Calling Chicken? Enchiladas	152	1.5
	Optional side dish/appetizer		
	Snack		
	Dinner		
	Mango-licious Barbecue Shrimp	390	5
	Optional side dish/appetizer		
	Snack		
	Total Calorie and Fat Intake from Main Courses:	**618**	**6.75**

The Sierras Solution
Menu Plan: Six Weeks
of Delicious, Satisfying,
Nutritious Meals for
Your Family

—

Week Six

		CALORIES	FAT GRAMS
Monday	**Breakfast**		
	AOS Taters and Eggs	158	0.1
	Lunch		
	Crabby Portobellos	148	0
	Optional side dish/appetizer		
	Snack		
	Dinner		
	Pork Chops au Poivre	167	4
	Optional side dish/appetizer		
	Snack		
	Total Calorie and Fat Intake from Main Courses:	**473**	**4.1**
Tuesday	**Breakfast**		
	Candy Apple Breakfast Pudding	208	1.5
	Lunch		
	Not Your Grandma's Chicken Salad Pita	189	2.6
	Optional side dish/appetizer		
	Snack		
	Dinner		
	Chicken Piccata	130	1.5
	Optional side dish/appetizer		
	Snack		
	Total Calorie and Fat Intake from Main Courses:	**527**	**5.6**
Wednesday	**Breakfast**		
	Huevos Rancheros Burritos	172	0
	Lunch		
	Very Veggie Stuffed Bell Peppers	165	7
	Optional side dish/appetizer		
	Snack		

The
Sierras
Solution
Eating
Plan
—
224

		CALORIES	FAT GRAMS
Wednesday	**Dinner**		
	Apple of My Eye Pork Stir-Fry	351	3
	Optional side dish/appetizer		
	Snack		
	Total Calorie and Fat Intake from Main Courses:	**688**	**10**
Thursday	**Breakfast**		
	Zenaida's Quiche	202	0
	Lunch		
	Parmesan-Encrusted Tilapia	235	4
	Optional side dish/appetizer		
	Snack		
	Dinner		
	Chicken Marsala	198	1.5
	Optional side dish/appetizer		
	Snack		
	Total Calorie and Fat Intake from Main Courses:	**641**	**7**
Friday	**Breakfast**		
	Mama Mia's Breakfast Calzone	110	0.5
	Lunch		
	Mandarin Chicken Wrap	151	1
	Optional side dish/appetizer		
	Snack		
	Dinner		
	Balsamic Baked Chicken	173	1.5
	Optional side dish/appetizer		
	Snack		
	Total Calorie and Fat Intake from Main Courses:	**434**	**3**
Saturday	**Breakfast**		
	Emu Scramble	146	2
	Lunch		
	Sweet Potato Couscous	204	1
	Optional side dish/appetizer		

The Sierras Solution Menu Plan: Six Weeks of Delicious, Satisfying, Nutritious Meals for Your Family

---

		CALORIES	FAT GRAMS
Saturday	**Snack**		
	Dinner		
	Reedley's Best Pizza	238	3
	Optional side dish/appetizer		
	Snack		
	Total Calorie and Fat Intake		
	from Main Courses:	**588**	**6**
Sunday	**Breakfast**		
	The Popeye Special Omelet	110	0.5
	Lunch		
	Happy as a Clam Pasta	238	2
	Optional side dish/appetizer		
	Snack		
	Dinner		
	Orange You Glad It's Scallops?	154	2
	Optional side dish/appetizer		
	Snack		
	Total Calorie and Fat Intake		
	from Main Courses:	**502**	**4.5**

The
Sierras
Solution
Eating
Plan

———

226

Chapter 12

The Sierras Solution Recipes: Decadent-Tasting Favorites Your Whole Family Will Love

Appetizers, Dips, and Sauces

All Choked Up Artichoke Dip

1 19-ounce can artichoke hearts, drained
¼ cup fat-free sour cream
¼ cup fat-free ricotta
¼ cup chopped scallions (about 1 bunch)
¼ cup chopped fresh flat-leaf parsley
3 tablespoons grated Parmesan
1 teaspoon minced garlic
3 tablespoons fat-free mayonnaise
Fat-free tortilla chips or cut-up vegetables, for serving

Place all ingredients in a food processor fitted with the blade attachment and process until slightly chunky. Avoid overprocessing—you don't want it puréed. Serve—either immediately at room temperature or chilled—with fat-free tortilla chips or vegetables.

SERVES 4: ¼ CUP PER PERSON
NUTRITION INFORMATION (PER SERVING): CALORIES: 74.8 FAT: 1 G
PROTEIN: 4.4 G

All Curried Up Dip/Spread

Nonfat cooking spray
1 cup minced sweet onion
1 tablespoon curry powder
2 cups fat-free ricotta
Salt and pepper to taste
Cut-up vegetables and pita wedges, for serving

Spray a medium skillet with nonfat cooking spray and heat over medium heat. Add onions and cook until they become translucent, about 3 minutes. Add the curry powder and cook 1 minute more. Pour into a medium bowl and let cool.

Stir the ricotta into the curry mixture. Season with salt and pepper. Chill for at least 1 hour and up to 3 days. Serve with fresh vegetables and pita wedges.

SERVES 8: ¼ CUP PER PERSON
NUTRITION INFORMATION (PER SERVING): CALORIES: 63 FAT: 0 G
PROTEIN: 8 G

All Steamed Up Artichokes

4 large artichokes
1 lemon, cut into quarters

Slice about an inch off the artichoke tops and trim the stems. Remove the smaller outer leaves at the bottom of the artichoke and trim any hard, spiky points with scissors. Be careful—the thorns can cause injury.

Place about 2 inches of water in the bottom pan of a double boiler/steamer and bring to a boil. (Feel free to use a steamer insert instead of a double boiler.) Once the steam starts to rise, place the artichokes in the top pan with holes, cover, and steam for 25 to 30 minutes, until the bottom is tender and the outer leaves can be pulled off easily.

Remove the artichokes from the pan and place them immediately into a large bowl of ice water. Drain and refrigerate until serving time.

The
Sierras
Solution
Eating
Plan

228

Serve on chilled plates with lemon wedges. You may use bottled fat-free Italian dressing as a dip or try the curry dip from the asparagus recipe below.

SERVES 4: 1 ARTICHOKE PER PERSON
NUTRITION INFORMATION (PER SERVING): CALORIES: 78 FAT: 0 G
PROTEIN: 5 G

Asparagus with Dip

2 pounds asparagus
½ cup fat-free mayonnaise
¼ teaspoon curry powder
2 garlic cloves, minced
Salt and pepper to taste

Cut or snap off the woody stems of the asparagus and rinse the asparagus well. Place on a microwave-safe plate and microwave until fork-tender, about 3 to 6 minutes, being careful not to overcook it. You might have to cook the asparagus in batches.

Take the asparagus out of the microwave and place in large bowl of ice water to stop the cooking process. Drain immediately.

In a small bowl, combine the mayonnaise, curry, garlic, salt, and pepper.

Place the asparagus in a fan shape on a large serving plate and serve, chilled or at room temperature, with the dip.

SERVES 6: ABOUT 7 SPEARS WITH DIP PER PERSON
NUTRITION INFORMATION (PER SERVING): CALORIES: 50 FAT: 0 G
PROTEIN: 4 G

Barbecue Sauce

1 cup ketchup
¼ cup Splenda brown sugar
¼ cup soy sauce

The Sierras
Solution Recipes:
Decadent-Tasting
Favorites Your Whole
Family Will Love
—

2 tablespoons Worcestershire sauce
¼ teaspoon chili powder
3 tablespoons cumin
Salt and pepper to taste

Place all ingredients in a small saucepan, stir, and cook 2 minutes over medium heat.

SERVES 4: ¼ CUP PER PERSON IF USED AS A DIP
NUTRITION INFORMATION (PER SERVING): CALORIES: 21.8 FAT: 0.2 G
PROTEIN: 0.6 G

Bruschetta, Anyone?

3 large tomatoes, seeded and chopped
1 large onion, minced
1 clove garlic, chopped
1 tablespoon chopped fresh basil
1 tablespoon chopped fresh oregano
¼ cup grated fat-free Parmesan
Salt and pepper to taste
1 French baguette
Nonfat cooking spray

Preheat oven to 375°F.

In a small mixing bowl, combine tomatoes, onion, garlic, basil, oregano, Parmesan, salt, and pepper. Mix well, cover, and refrigerate.

Cut the baguette into 12 slices on the diagonal. Spray a baking sheet with nonfat cooking spray. Arrange the bread on the baking sheet and toast in the oven until golden brown. Remove from the oven. Reduce the heat to 250°F.

Spoon equal amounts of the mixture onto the toasted slices of bread. Place back in the oven for 5 minutes, until mixture is heated through.

Serve warm or at room temperature.

SERVES 6: 2 SLICES PER PERSON
NUTRITION INFORMATION (PER SERVING): CALORIES: 178 FAT: 1.4 G
PROTEIN: 1.4 G

The
Sierras
Solution
Eating
Plan

———

230

Crispy Panko Shrimp Appetizers

> 1 pound large (12 to 14 count) shrimp, peeled and
>   deveined
> ¼ cup cornstarch
> ¼ cup egg whites or Egg Beaters
> 1½ cups panko (Japanese breadcrumbs)
> 1 tablespoon seasoning salt (preferably Lawry's)
> White pepper to taste
> Nonfat cooking spray

Preheat the broiler. Place rack on second rung from the top.

Combine shrimp and cornstarch in a plastic bag. Seal and shake to coat.

In a medium bowl, whisk egg whites until foamy.

In another medium bowl, combine breadcrumbs, seasoning salt, and white pepper.

Dip shrimp into egg whites and then dredge in crumb mixture.

Place the shrimp on a baking sheet coated with nonfat cooking spray. Lightly spray the shrimp with nonfat spray.

Broil 6 minutes or until shrimp are done, turning once after 3 minutes. Serve with cocktail sauce.

SERVES 6 TO 7: 2 SHRIMP PER PERSON
NUTRITION INFORMATION (PER SERVING): CALORIES: 106 FAT: 1.5 G
PROTEIN: 13 G

Fall Fruit with Vanilla-Maple Dip

> 2 cups fat-free vanilla yogurt
> ½ cup light or sugar-free maple syrup
> 1 large apple (any kind)
> 1 large pear
> 2 tablespoons fresh-squeezed lemon juice
> 1 pound green grapes

Combine yogurt and maple syrup in a small bowl. Chill for at least 1 hour.

Core and slice the pear and apple. Sprinkle with lemon juice to prevent the fruit from turning brown. Wash the grapes.

The Sierras
Solution Recipes:
Decadent-Tasting
Favorites Your Whole
Family Will Love

———

Arrange the fruit decoratively on a large platter and place a small bowl of dip in the center.

SERVES 8: ¼ CUP YOGURT PER PERSON
NUTRITION INFORMATION (PER SERVING): CALORIES: 79 FAT: 0 G
PROTEIN: 3 G

Fine Herb Sauce

*½ cup cooking sherry (or fat-free chicken, beef, or vegetable
  stock)*
2 tablespoons minced fresh thyme
2 tablespoons minced fresh basil
2 tablespoons minced fresh oregano
Salt and pepper

This is a good sauce for sautéed chicken, pork, or beef.

Once meat has been sautéed, remove it from the pan and set aside, keeping it warm.

Combine sherry and ½ cup water.

Remove pan from heat, pour off excess fat, and deglaze the pan with sherry mixture, stirring to remove browned bits of food from the bottom. Reduce mixture by half.

Add the herbs, salt, and pepper and simmer for 2 minutes.

Slice meat and cover with herb sauce. Serve immediately.

SERVES 4: ⅛ CUP PER PERSON
NUTRITION INFORMATION (PER SERVING): CALORIES: 49.5 FAT: 0.3 G
PROTEIN: 0.4 G

The
Sierras
Solution
Eating
Plan

———

232

Mexican Spring Rolls

1 pound chicken tenders
2 cups orange juice
¼ cup fresh-squeezed lime juice

¼ cup minced fresh cilantro

1 tablespoon cumin

Salt and pepper to taste

½ cup peeled jicama, cut into thin strips

1 4-ounce can chopped green chilies

¼ cup diced scallions

12 round 8-inch rice papers (available in Asian specialty section of supermarket)

Combine the chicken and orange juice in a medium skillet and bring to a simmer over medium heat. Reduce the heat to low and simmer until cooked through, 7 to 9 minutes. Drain the chicken, transfer to a plate, and discard the orange juice.

Let stand until cool enough to handle. Cut the chicken into thin strips and set aside.

Meanwhile, combine the lime juice, cilantro, cumin, salt, and pepper in a medium bowl. Add chicken and toss to coat. Set aside.

Fill a shallow dish with warm water. Working with one rice paper at a time, dip into water and soak until softened, 20 to 30 seconds. Transfer the rice paper to a piece of damp paper towel. Across the lower third of a rice paper sheet, top with 4 strips of chicken, 1 tablespoon of jicama, and 1 teaspoon each of green chilies and scallion. Leave a ¼-inch margin on each side. Fold the bottom of the rice paper over the filling, fold in the sides, and roll up tightly. Transfer to a large plate. Cover with a damp towel. Repeat the process with the remaining sheets of rice paper and filling.

SERVES 12: 1 SPRING ROLL PER PERSON

NUTRITION INFORMATION (PER SERVING): CALORIES: 45 FAT: 1 G

PROTEIN: 3 G

No Crying Onion Quesadillas

Nonfat cooking spray

1 large Vidalia or sweet onion, peeled and cut into ¼-inch slices

1 jalapeño pepper

The Sierras
Solution Recipes:
Decadent-Tasting
Favorites Your Whole
Family Will Love

———

233

4 7-inch fat-free flour tortillas
¾ cup grated fat-free mozzarella or fat-free Monterey Jack
¼ cup minced fresh cilantro
Salsa or fat-free sour cream, for serving

Preheat oven to 375°F or preheat a grill to medium high heat. Spray a cookie sheet with nonfat cooking spray if using the oven.

Arrange onion slices and jalapeño on a cookie sheet, or if grilling place them directly on the grill. Roast until onions and jalapeño start to brown, or if grilling until lightly charred and softened.

Place cooked onions in a bowl, separating into rings. Place the jalapeño in a small bowl and cover with foil or plastic wrap. This will steam the skin, which you can simply remove by rubbing it off. After removing the skin, slice open the jalapeño, remove the seeds, then dice. Wear gloves when handling jalapeños.

Take 2 tortillas and divide the onion, jalapeño, cheese, and cilantro between them. Cover with the remaining 2 tortillas.

Spray a medium skillet with nonfat cooking spray and heat over medium heat. With a spatula, transfer quesadillas to skillet and cook for 3 to 4 minutes, or until the bottom tortillas turn a golden brown.

Lightly spray the top tortillas with nonfat cooking spray. Using two spatulas, sandwich the quesadillas between them and flip over to brown the other side.

Transfer quesadillas to a cutting board and cut into wedges. Serve immediately with salsa or fat-free sour cream, if desired.

SERVES 2: 1 QUESADILLA PER PERSON
NUTRITION INFORMATION (PER SERVING): CALORIES: 109.5 FAT: 3.2 G
PROTEIN: 4.2 G

The
Sierras
Solution
Eating
Plan
———
234

No-Fry Sweet Potato French Fries

Nonfat cooking spray
2 large sweet potatoes, cut lengthwise into ½-inch strips
1 teaspoon chili powder
½ cup grated fat-free Parmesan

1 teaspoon cayenne pepper
Salt to taste

Preheat oven to 450°F.

Spray a large baking sheet with nonfat spray.

Place sweet potatoes fries into a large bowl and spray with nonfat cooking spray, tossing to coat. This helps the spices to adhere.

Add the chili powder, Parmesan, and cayenne pepper. Toss to coat well.

Arrange fries on a baking sheet in single layer. Bake 30 to 35 minutes, turning the fries over halfway through.

Season with salt.

SERVES 4: ABOUT 12 FRIES PER PERSON
NUTRITION INFORMATION (PER SERVING): CALORIES: 74 FAT: 1 G
PROTEIN: 4 G

Roasted Garlic Hummus

2 whole garlic bulbs
Nonfat cooking spray
¼ cup chopped red onion
2 8-ounce cans garbanzo beans, drained
1 tablespoon chopped fresh flat-leaf parsley
1 teaspoon cayenne pepper
1 tablespoon fresh-squeezed lemon juice
Salt and pepper to taste

Preheat the oven to 425°F.

Slice off the tops of the garlic bulbs, making sure not to cut the root ends. Cut deep enough to expose most of the cloves.

Line a cookie sheet or small baking dish with foil for easy cleanup, add the garlic, and spray with nonfat cooking spray.

Place in the oven and cook for 45 minutes, until the garlic is completely soft and lightly browned. Let the garlic cool and then squeeze it out of the husk.

In a food processor fitted with the blade attachment or a blender, add

The Sierras
Solution Recipes:
Decadent-Tasting
Favorites Your Whole
Family Will Love

——

235

the garlic and onions and pulse until finely blended. Add garbanzo beans, one can at a time, and pulse to purée. Add the parsley, cayenne pepper, lemon juice, salt, and pepper, pulsing until mixture is smooth.

Serve warm or chilled.

SERVES 8: ¼ CUP PER PERSON
NUTRITION INFORMATION (PER SERVING): CALORIES: 39 FAT: 0.3 G
PROTEIN: 1.4 G

South of the Border Dip

    1 cup fat-free refried beans
    ¾ teaspoon minced garlic
    ¾ teaspoon cumin
    ¾ teaspoon chili powder
    2 teaspoons fresh-squeezed lime juice
    Salt and pepper to taste
    ⅓ cup diced tomato
    ⅓ cup diced red onion
    ⅓ cup diced red bell pepper
    Fat-free tortilla chips or pita chips, for serving

In a blender or food processor fitted with the blade attachment, combine the beans, garlic, cumin, chili powder, lime juice, salt, and pepper. Pulse until mixture is smooth and creamy.

In a small bowl, combine the tomatoes, red onion, and red pepper. Add the bean mixture and stir until completely blended.

This dip may be served at room temperature or warm. To warm, microwave on high for 2 minutes, stirring after 1 minute, until the dip is heated through. Serve with fat-free tortilla or pita chips.

SERVES 6: ¼ CUP PER PERSON
NUTRITION INFORMATION (PER SERVING): CALORIES: 51.8 FAT: 0.3 G
PROTEIN: 2.5 G

The
Sierras
Solution
Eating
Plan

—

236

Southwestern Cheese Dip

8 ounces fat-free cream cheese
1 red bell pepper
1 yellow bell pepper
1 or 2 jalapeño peppers
½ teaspoon chili powder
Fat-free tortilla chips or cut-up vegetables, for serving
½ teaspoon garlic salt
2 tablespoons cumin

Remove cream cheese from package, place in bowl, and let it soften to room temperature.

Place red, yellow, and jalapeño peppers on a stovetop grill or place approximately 4 inches under a broiler. Char until skin is blackened. Place peppers in a medium bowl and cover with foil or plastic wrap. Let steam for at least 10 minutes.

Remove the charred skin by rubbing it off the peppers, wearing gloves to handle the jalapeño. Remove seeds from the inside of the peppers, dice, and set aside.

Once the cream cheese has softened, add the peppers, chili powder, garlic salt, and cumin. Mix thoroughly.

Chill for at least 1 hour.

Serve with fat-free tortilla chips and vegetables. This dip is also excellent as a sandwich spread.

SERVES 4: ¼ CUP PER PERSON
NUTRITION INFORMATION (PER SERVING): CALORIES: 65.5 FAT: 0 G
PROTEIN: 8.5 G

Spinach Dip

5 ounces fresh spinach (about half of a standard package)
½ cup fat-free plain yogurt
¾ cup fat-free cream cheese

The Sierras
Solution Recipes:
Decadent-Tasting
Favorites Your Whole
Family Will Love

—

½ teaspoon minced garlic
2 tablespoons chopped fresh flat-leaf parsley
2 tablespoons grated Parmesan
Salt and pepper to taste

Wash spinach well and shake off excess water. In a sauté pan, cook the spinach until wilted; squeeze out excess water from wilted leaves.

In food processor fitted with the blade attachment, add spinach, yogurt, cream cheese, garlic, parsley, Parmesan, salt, and pepper. Pulse until combined, but avoid overprocessing—you don't want it puréed.

You may prepare this up to a day in advance. Serve chilled or at room temperature with vegetables or fat-free pita chips. The dip also works well when served in a small, hollowed-out round bread. Save the bread you remove from the middle, to use along with vegetables for dipping.

SERVES 6: ¼ CUP PER PERSON
NUTRITION INFORMATION (PER SERVING): CALORIES: 56.8 FAT: 0.5 G
PROTEIN: 7 G

Sweet and Spicy Turkey Pinwheels

4 ounces fat-free cream cheese, softened to room
* temperature*
⅓ cup canned mandarin oranges, chopped and drained
1 tablespoon cumin
Salt and pepper to taste
4 10-inch fat-free flour tortillas
¼ cup diced scallions, green part only
6 ounces low-fat or fat-free smoked turkey, thinly sliced
½ cup spinach leaves, washed and stemmed

In medium bowl, combine the cream cheese, oranges, cumin, salt, and pepper, mixing well.

Lay out all of the flour tortillas and spread each with ¼ of the cream cheese mix. Be sure to leave a 1½-inch margin around the edges free of toppings.

The
Sierras
Solution
Eating
Plan

—

238

Sprinkle with scallions, then layer on turkey and spinach leaves. Roll tortillas tightly.

Slice the ends off and discard, then slice each tortilla into 6 pieces and lay on its side to form pinwheels.

You can make these one or two days in advance, but if cutting pinwheels, do not refrigerate more than 8 hours before eating.

SERVES 6: 4 PINWHEELS PER PERSON
NUTRITION INFORMATION (PER SERVING): CALORIES: 42 FAT: 1 G
PROTEIN: 4 G

Up in Smoke Turkey Spread

> 8 ounces fat-free cream cheese, softened to room
>   temperature
> 8 ounces smoked turkey, sliced or cubed
> ¼ cup chopped fresh cilantro
> ¼ teaspoon cayenne pepper
> Salt and pepper to taste

In a food processor fitted with the blade attachment, add the cream cheese, turkey, and cilantro. Pulse until mixture is smooth, but do not overprocess. Add the cayenne pepper, salt, and pepper. Pulse until incorporated.

Chill for at least 1 hour.

Serve with fat-free tortilla chips and vegetables. This dip is also excellent as a sandwich spread.

SERVES 4: ¼ CUP PER PERSON
NUTRITION INFORMATION (PER SERVING): CALORIES: 115 FAT: 1.5 G
PROTEIN: 18 G

Wild Mushroom Crostini

> 1 French baguette
> Nonfat cooking spray
> 2 shallots, diced

The Sierras
Solution Recipes:
Decadent-Tasting
Favorites Your Whole
Family Will Love

—

239

1 cup sliced cremini mushrooms
½ cup sliced shiitake mushrooms
¼ cup fat-free cream cheese, softened to room temperature
1 tablespoon fresh thyme
Salt and pepper to taste

Preheat oven to 350°F.

Cut the bread into 16 slices on the diagonal. Arrange the slices on a baking sheet and toast in the oven until golden brown, 6 to 8 minutes. Remove from the oven and set aside.

Spray a large skillet with nonfat cooking spray. Add shallots and sauté until tender over medium heat.

Add mushrooms to skillet and sauté until moist and tender.

Place mushroom sauté into food processor fitted with the blade attachment and pulse until mushrooms are finely chopped. Set aside.

In a medium bowl, add cream cheese, thyme, and mushrooms. Mix until blended. Season with salt and pepper and stir to combine.

Spread mushroom mixture evenly onto crostini and serve immediately.

The spread keeps for up to 3 days tightly covered in the refrigerator. Before serving, allow to return to room temperature.

SERVES 16: 1 SLICE WITH 2 TABLESPOONS OF SPREAD
NUTRITION INFORMATION (PER SERVING): CALORIES: 74 FAT: 0 G
PROTEIN: 84 G

Zucchini Fingers

½ cup egg whites or Egg Beaters
1 cup panko (Japanese breadcrumbs)
¼ cup grated fat-free Parmesan
2 tablespoons seasoning salt (preferably Lawry's)
1 teaspoon black pepper
4 small zucchini
Nonfat cooking spray

The
Sierras
Solution
Eating
Plan
———
240

Preheat oven to 450°F.

Place egg whites in a small bowl and beat lightly.

In separate bowl, add panko, Parmesan, salt, and pepper.

Cut the zucchini into quarters lengthwise, dip into egg whites to coat thoroughly, then dip into breadcrumb mixture.

Spray a cookie sheet with nonfat cooking spray. Arrange zucchini fingers on the cookie sheet and cook for 18 to 25 minutes, until golden brown and tender. Serve immediately.

SERVES 4: 4 ZUCCHINI FINGERS PER PERSON
NUTRITION INFORMATION (PER SERVING): CALORIES: 119 FAT: 1.5 G
PROTEIN: 8 G

Breakfast

All Wrapped Up

2 8-inch fat-free tortillas
2 slices turkey bacon
¼ cup chopped sweet red pepper
Salt and pepper to taste
½ cup egg whites or Egg Beaters
¼ cup chopped tomato
Salsa or nonfat sour cream, for serving

Wrap the tortillas in foil and warm briefly in the oven according to the package directions.

In a medium skillet, cook turkey bacon until brown and crispy. Remove bacon from skillet, blot dry on a paper towel, chop, and return to the skillet.

Add red pepper, salt, and pepper to the skillet and cook for 3 minutes.

Add egg whites and cook, stirring, for 2 minutes, until egg begins to set. Remove skillet from heat, add tomatoes, and stir.

Spoon mixture into warmed tortilla, then roll tortilla around filling. Serve immediately.

The Sierras
Solution Recipes:
Decadent-Tasting
Favorites Your Whole
Family Will Love

———

Serves 4: 1 wrap per person
Nutrition Information (per serving): Calories: 177 Fat: 1 g
Protein: 10 g

AOS Breakfast Stacker

Nonfat cooking spray
Salt and pepper to taste
½ cup egg whites or Egg Beaters
4 English muffins
4 slices fat-free American cheese
4 slices thin-sliced turkey bacon

Preheat oven to 325°F.

Spray a muffin pan with nonfat cooking spray.

Add salt and pepper to egg whites and beat lightly. Pour equal amounts of egg whites into four of the muffin slots.

Place in oven and cook until set, 6 to 8 minutes.

Separate the English muffins, using a fork. Toast.

As soon as you pull the muffins from the toaster, place a single slice of cheese on one muffin half.

On a microwave-safe plate, heat turkey bacon slices in microwave for 1 to 2 minutes on high. Remove bacon and place on top of the melted cheese.

Remove egg whites from the oven. Pop out eggs and place on top of turkey bacon. Serve immediately.

Serves 4: 1 breakfast sandwich per person
Nutritional Information (per serving): Calories: 200 Fat: 2 g
Protein: 11 g

AOS Taters and Eggs

2 medium russet potatoes
Nonfat cooking spray
Salt and pepper to taste

The
Sierras
Solution
Eating
Plan

242

1 cup egg whites or Egg Beaters
1 bunch chives, chopped
½ cup shredded fat-free cheddar cheese
Salsa or fat-free sour cream, for serving

Wash potatoes and pat dry. Place potatoes in the microwave and cook on high until you can easily insert and remove a knife, about 8 to 12 minutes.

Spray a skillet with nonfat cooking spray and heat over medium heat.

Add salt and pepper to egg whites and beat lightly. Pour into the skillet and scramble, making sure to remove pan from heat once the eggs are nearly done. Add the chives and continue cooking eggs until firm, using residual heat from the pan.

Remove potatoes from the microwave and slice in half lengthwise. Scoop out the inside of each potato into a bowl. The skin is now your boat.

Mash the potato in the bowl, seasoning to taste. Add egg white–chive mixture and stir.

Divide into four portions and top with cheddar cheese.

Serve immediately with salsa or fat-free sour cream if desired.

SERVES 4: ½ CUP PER PERSON
NUTRITION INFORMATION (PER SERVING): CALORIES: 158 FAT: 0.1 G
PROTEIN: 23 G

Candy Apple Breakfast Pudding

2 large Granny Smith apples
¾ teaspoon ground cinnamon
¼ cup Splenda brown sugar
½ cup light corn syrup
Nonfat cooking spray
10 ½-inch-thick slices of French or Italian bread
¼ cup egg whites or Egg Beaters
1¼ cups fat-free milk
1 teaspoon vanilla extract
¼ teaspoon ground allspice

The Sierras
Solution Recipes:
Decadent-Tasting
Favorites Your Whole
Family Will Love

—

243

Peel, core, and slice the apples. You should have 2 cups.

Place apples in a small saucepan with ¼ cup water and bring to a boil. Reduce heat, and cook over medium low heat for 6 to 8 minutes, until apples are tender.

Drain apples in a colander and put into a small bowl. Add cinnamon and stir gently. Set aside.

In small saucepan, combine the brown sugar and corn syrup. Bring mixture to a boil over medium heat while stirring. Remove from heat.

Spray a 2-quart square baking dish with nonfat cooking spray, then pour in brown sugar mixture.

Arrange 5 of the bread slices in a layer on top of the caramel mixture in the baking dish, trimming bread to fit.

Spoon cooked apples evenly over bread layer. Arrange the remaining bread slices on top.

In a medium mixing bowl, combine the eggs, milk, vanilla, and allspice. Carefully pour the egg mixture over the bread, pressing down to moisten the bread slices completely.

Cover with plastic wrap and refrigerate for at least 2½ hours or up to 24 hours.

When you are ready to serve, preheat the oven to 325°F. Remove plastic wrap and bake, uncovered, for 45 minutes, until a knife inserted in the center comes out clean.

Remove from oven and run a clean knife around the edges to loosen. Let stand for 15 minutes.

Invert the pudding onto a platter that is larger than the square baking dish. Spoon the remaining brown sugar sauce over the pudding. Cut into rectangles or squares and serve warm or cool.

SERVES 6: 6 OUNCES PER PERSON
NUTRITION INFORMATION (PER SERVING): CALORIES: 208 FAT: 1.5 G
PROTEIN: 5 G

The
Sierras
Solution
Eating
Plan
—
244

Emu Scramble

Nonfat cooking spray
1 cup egg whites or Egg Beaters

Salt and pepper to taste
2 ounces Canadian bacon, chopped
¼ cup fat-free cheddar cheese
¼ cup chopped tomatoes
2 tablespoons chopped scallions

Spray a large skillet with nonfat spray and heat over medium high heat.

Once pan is heated, add eggs, salt, pepper, Canadian bacon, and cheddar cheese. Stir until eggs start to come together.

Just before eggs are completely cooked, remove the pan from heat.

Stir in the tomatoes and scallions. Let the residual heat from the pan continue to cook the eggs the rest of the way. Serve immediately.

SERVES 2: ½ CUP PER PERSON

NUTRITION INFORMATION (PER SERVING): CALORIES: 146 FAT: 2 G
PROTEIN: 23 G

Huevos Rancheros Burritos

2 10-inch fat-free flour tortillas
Nonfat cooking spray
1 cup egg whites or Egg Beaters
2 tablespoons minced fresh cilantro
Salt and pepper to taste
¼ cup shredded fat-free cheddar cheese
¼ cup medium salsa

Wrap the tortillas in foil and warm briefly in the oven according to package directions.

Spray a skillet with nonfat cooking spray and heat over medium heat.

In a small mixing bowl, combine egg whites, cilantro, salt, and pepper. Beat lightly with a fork to combine.

Add egg mixture to skillet and cook just until eggs start to set. Remove the pan from heat and continue cooking eggs with the residual heat from the pan.

Divide the egg mixture evenly between the tortillas. Top with cheese and salsa, evenly distributed.

The Sierras
Solution Recipes:
Decadent-Tasting
Favorites Your Whole
Family Will Love

—

Fold up tortillas over filling, tucking in the ends like an envelope. Serve immediately.

SERVES 2: 1 BURRITO PER PERSON
NUTRITION INFORMATION (PER SERVING): CALORIES: 172 FAT: 0 G
PROTEIN: 15 G

Mama Mia's Breakfast Calzone

1 pound (4 loaves) frozen French bread dough, thawed
Nonfat cooking spray
⅛ teaspoon minced garlic
¼ cup chopped sweet onion
½ cup chopped white button mushrooms
¼ cup egg whites or Egg Beaters
1 cup shredded fat-free mozzarella
1 tablespoon chopped fresh basil
Black pepper to taste

Remove individual dough loaves from package and roll, following package directions.

Spray a medium skillet with nonfat cooking spray; add garlic and sauté briefly until you can smell the garlic. Add onions and sauté until translucent. Add mushrooms and cook until tender. Drain and cool. Set aside.

Add egg whites, cheese, basil, and pepper to mushroom mixture. Mix well.

Roll each loaf into a 16 × 12-inch square. Spread half of the mushroom mixture on each loaf, leaving a 1-inch margin all around. Roll jelly-roll style, starting at the narrow (short) end. Seal edges with water. Place on a baking sheet that has been sprayed with nonfat spray. Cover and refrigerate overnight.

The next morning, preheat the oven to 350°F. Bake for 25 minutes. To make calzones golden brown, brush tops with a little egg white and bake 5 to 10 minutes more.

The
Sierras
Solution
Eating
Plan

——

246

SERVES 4: 1 CALZONE PER PERSON
NUTRITION INFORMATION (PER SERVING): CALORIES: 110 FAT: 0.5 G
PROTEIN: 18 G

Oh, My, Oatmeal Bake

2 cups uncooked quick-cooking oats
½ cup Splenda brown sugar
⅓ cup raisins
1 teaspoon baking powder
1½ cups fat-free milk
½ cup applesauce
¼ cup egg whites or Egg Beaters
Nonfat cooking spray

Preheat oven to 375°F.

In a medium mixing bowl, combine oats, brown sugar, raisins, and baking powder.

In a small mixing bowl, combine milk, applesauce, and egg whites.

Add milk mixture to oat mixture. Stir well.

Spray an 8-inch-square baking dish with nonfat cooking spray. Pour oat mixture in, and bake for 20 minutes. Serve warm.

SERVES 5: ⅔ CUP PER PERSON
NUTRITION INFORMATION (PER SERVING): CALORIES: 103 FAT: 0.8 G
PROTEIN: 4 G

The Popeye Special Omelet

6 tablespoons egg whites or Egg Beaters
2 teaspoons chopped fresh dill (or any other herb)
Salt and pepper to taste
Nonfat cooking spray
¼ cup baby spinach leaves
1 plum tomato, diced
2 tablespoons grated fat-free cheddar cheese

In a medium mixing bowl, whisk egg whites, dill, salt, and pepper together until soft peaks form.

The Sierras
Solution Recipes:
Decadent-Tasting
Favorites Your Whole
Family Will Love

——

247

Spray a small skillet or omelet pan with nonfat cooking spray and heat over medium heat.

Pour egg mixture into the pan and stir until eggs begin to set. Remove pan from heat.

Using the handle as your guide, picture creating a cross, with your handle being the vertical part of the cross. Add the spinach, tomatoes, and cheddar cheese horizontally across in the middle of your pan.

Tilt the pan up and place your spatula under the omelet at the base of the handle. Fold the omelet away from you. Once the omelet is completely folded, place it on plate and serve immediately.

SERVES 1

NUTRITION INFORMATION (PER SERVING): CALORIES: 110 FAT: 0.5 G
PROTEIN: 18 G

Sierra Blueberry Pancakes

1 cup plus 2 tablespoons whole-wheat flour
1 tablespoon Splenda brown sugar
1½ teaspoons baking powder
⅛ teaspoon salt
2 tablespoons applesauce
1 cup plus 2 tablespoons water or fat-free milk
½ cup fresh or frozen blueberries or other fruit, such as
    sliced bananas or peaches
Nonfat cooking spray

In a medium bowl, mix all dry ingredients together.

Add applesauce and water. The batter should drip from the spoon, but should not be runny. Take half of the blueberries and smash them together, allowing the juices to run out. Add them to the mix. This will help flavor the batter and will turn the batter a light purple. Add the remaining whole blueberries.

Spray a griddle or frying pan with nonfat cooking spray and heat over medium heat.

Ladle ¼ cup of batter into the pan and let it cook until small bubbles

The
Sierras
Solution
Eating
Plan

———

248

form in the center and/or the edges are dry. Flip pancake over and cook for an additional minute or two.

Serve immediately.

SERVES 3: 2 PANCAKES PER PERSON
NUTRITION INFORMATION (PER SERVING): CALORIES: 152 FAT: 0.5 G
PROTEIN: 4 G

Sorry, Charlie, Breakfast Melt

5 ounces fat-free cream cheese
2 tablespoons diced pimentos
1 tablespoon capers
1 tablespoon Old Bay Seasoning
Salt and pepper to taste
1 6½-ounce can light tuna packed in water, drained
3 English muffins, split and toasted
1 large tomato, cut into 6 slices

Preheat the broiler.

In a small bowl, combine cream cheese, pimentos, and capers, mixing thoroughly.

Add Old Bay Seasoning, salt, and pepper and mix until incorporated. Set aside.

In a separate bowl, combine ⅓ of the cream-cheese mixture with the tuna. Spread the mixture over each of the split muffin halves, dividing evenly.

Place broiler rack on the second rung from the top and broil for about 3 minutes, until heated through. Remove from oven.

Top each split muffin half with the tomato slices, then divide the remaining cheese spread evenly over each half. Return to the broiler until the cheese spread melts, about 1 minute.

SERVES 3: TWO HALVES PER PERSON
NUTRITION INFORMATION (PER SERVING): CALORIES: 265 FAT: 3 G
PROTEIN: 24 G

The Sierras
Solution Recipes:
Decadent-Tasting
Favorites Your Whole
Family Will Love
—

Zenaida's Quiche

Nonfat cooking spray
¾ cup egg whites or Egg Beaters
1 cup fat-free evaporated milk
⅓ cup all-purpose flour
1½ cups shredded fat-free cheddar cheese
1½ cups shredded fat-free mozzarella
1 8-ounce can green chilies, chopped
½ cup chunky medium salsa, drained, plus additional salsa
  for serving
Salt and pepper to taste
Fat-free sour cream, for serving

Preheat the oven to 350°F.

Spray an 8- or 9-inch glass pie plate with nonfat cooking spray.

In a medium bowl, combine egg whites, milk, flour, salt, and pepper. Beat well until smooth.

Add ¼ cup of each cheese and green chilies into milk mixture, stirring to combine. Reserve the remaining cheese for the topping.

Spoon a small amount of drained salsa on the bottom of the pie plate and spread around. This will help keep the quiche from sticking.

Ladle half of the cheese and milk mixture over the salsa. Spoon the remaining salsa over this layer, then top with remaining cheese-milk mixture.

Bake for 30 to 35 minutes, until set and puffy.

Top with the reserved cheese and bake an additional 5 minutes until melted.

Serve with additional salsa and fat-free sour cream if desired.

The
Sierras
Solution
Eating
Plan

———

250

SERVES 6: 1 SLICE (APPROXIMATELY 6 OUNCES) PER PERSON

NUTRITION INFORMATION (PER SERVING): CALORIES: 202 FAT: 0 G

PROTEIN: 15 G

Lunch

Apricot Ginger Pita

1 16-ounce pork tenderloin
Seasoning salt (preferably Lawry's) to taste
2 cups shredded romaine lettuce
½ cup crumbled fat-free feta
8 fat-free pitas
1 cup apricot preserves
2 tablespoons soy sauce
1 tablespoon minced fresh ginger

Preheat a grill or the broiler.

Season pork tenderloin with seasoning salt.

Grill or broil the tenderloin until its internal temperature reaches 160° to 165°F, 15 to 18 minutes.

Remove tenderloin from heat and let it sit for at least 5 minutes before slicing.

In a small saucepan, add apricot preserves and heat slowly over low heat until the preserves liquefy. Add soy sauce and fresh ginger and stir to combine. Set aside to cool.

In a medium bowl, add shredded lettuce and toss with the apricot ginger sauce.

Take 1 pita and divide in half. Add ¼ cup of lettuce to each half, followed by 1½ teaspoons of feta in each half. Top with 2 ounces of sliced pork tenderloin. Repeat with remaining pitas.

Serve immediately.

SERVES 8: 1 PITA PER PERSON
NUTRITION INFORMATION (PER SERVING): CALORIES: 190.1 FAT: 1.3 G
PROTEIN: 18 G

The Sierras
Solution Recipes:
Decadent-Tasting
Favorites Your Whole
Family Will Love

———

Crabby Portobellos

8 *portobello mushrooms, each approximately 4 inches in
diameter*
8 *ounces fat-free cream cheese, softened to room
temperature*
½ *cup diced scallion tops (green part only)*
1 *teaspoon lemon juice*
¼ *cup fat-free mayonnaise*
1 *teaspoon Old Bay Seasoning*
1 *pound lump canned crabmeat*
½ *cup diced jarred roasted red peppers*
½ *cup shredded fat-free mozzarella*
½ *cup fat-free breadcrumbs*
Salt and pepper to taste

Preheat oven to 425°F.

Remove and discard the brown gills from the undersides of the mushrooms, using a spoon. Remove and discard the stems. Set mushrooms aside.

Using a handheld electric mixer, beat cream cheese until smooth. Add scallion tops, lemon juice, mayonnaise, and Old Bay Seasoning. Mix until well blended.

Place cheese mixture in a large bowl and stir in crabmeat, red peppers and mozzarella.

Spoon mixture evenly into mushroom caps, and sprinkle each cap with 1 tablespoon breadcrumbs. Place on an unsprayed baking sheet.

Bake for 15 minutes or until tops are lightly browned. Serve immediately.

The
Sierras
Solution
Eating
Plan

———

252

SERVES 8: 1 MUSHROOM PER PERSON
NUTRITION INFORMATION (PER SERVING): CALORIES: 148 FAT: 0 G
PROTEIN: 21 G

Crispy Crisp Chicken Fingers

4 4-ounce skinless, boneless chicken breasts
½ cup egg whites or Egg Beaters
1½ cups panko (Japanese breadcrumbs)
2 tablespoons seasoning salt (preferably Lawry's)
1 teaspoon black pepper
Nonfat cooking spray

Preheat oven to 450°F.
Cut each chicken breast into 6 strips.
Add egg whites to a small mixing bowl and beat lightly.
In separate small bowl, add panko, seasoning salt, and pepper.
Dip strips into egg whites and coat thoroughly, then dip into bread-crumb mixture.
Spray a baking sheet with nonfat cooking spray. Place strips on baking sheet and bake for 8 to 10 minutes, turning after 4 minutes, until golden brown. Serve immediately.

SERVES 4: 6 STRIPS PER PERSON
NUTRITION INFORMATION (PER SERVING): CALORIES: 176 FAT: 1.5 G
PROTEIN: 34.5 G

Hakuna Matata Frittata

1½ cups egg whites or Egg Beaters
¼ cup fat-free milk
Salt and pepper to taste
1 cup cooked and diced white-meat chicken
1 cup sliced white button mushrooms
2 tablespoons thinly sliced scallions
Nonfat cooking spray
¼ cup shredded fat-free cheddar cheese

The Sierras
Solution Recipes:
Decadent-Tasting
Favorites Your Whole
Family Will Love

———

253

In a small mixing bowl, stir together egg whites, milk, salt, and pepper. Set aside.

In a medium mixing bowl, combine chicken, mushrooms, and scallions.

Spray an ovenproof skillet with nonfat cooking spray and heat over medium low heat. Add egg mixture and cook. As eggs set, run a spatula around the edge, lifting to allow the uncooked portion to flow underneath. Cook until eggs are almost set but the surface is still moist.

Press chicken mixture into the top of the egg mixture.

Place skillet under broiler 4 to 5 inches from heating element, and heat for 1 to 2 minutes, or until set. Top with cheese and continue cooking until cheese melts.

Cut frittata into 4 slices and serve immediately.

SERVES 4: 1 SLICE PER PERSON
NUTRITION INFORMATION (PER SERVING): CALORIES: 147 FAT: 1.5 G
PROTEIN: 16 G

Kickin' Chicken Wrap

4 4-ounce boneless, skinless chicken breasts
1 red onion, peeled and sliced thick
¾ teaspoon cumin
¾ teaspoon chili powder
Salt and pepper to taste
½ cup Barbecue Sauce (see page 229)
½ cup Southwestern Cheese Dip (see page 237)
4 fat-free or low-fat flour tortilla wraps
8 ounces fresh spinach leaves

The
Sierras
Solution
Eating
Plan

—

254

Preheat a grill or the broiler.

Season the chicken and the onion slices with cumin, chili powder, salt, and pepper.

Grill or broil the chicken until juices run clear, about 4 minutes per side. Grill the onion until it starts to caramelize.

Baste the chicken and onion with Barbecue Sauce and cook for another 3 minutes, remembering to baste each side. Remove from heat and let sit for at least 5 minutes before cutting the chicken into strips and dicing the onion.

Spread Southwestern Cheese Dip on each tortilla wrap. Place 4 ounces of sliced chicken strips in the center of each tortilla horizontally.

Add the onion and spinach leaves to the tortillas, distributing evenly. Roll tortilla and serve immediately.

SERVES 4: 1 TORTILLA PER PERSON
NUTRITION INFORMATION (PER SERVING): CALORIES: 302 FAT: 2 G
PROTEIN: 9 G

Mandarin Chicken Wraps

4 4-ounce boneless, skinless chicken breasts
1 cup shredded romaine lettuce
½ cup canned mandarin orange segments, drained
¼ cup prepared fat-free ginger dressing, such as Paul Newman's
4 fat-free whole-wheat tortilla wraps

Place chicken in a 4-quart stockpot and add water to cover. Bring to a boil, then lower heat to a simmer and cook until chicken is done, 18 to 20 minutes. Drain chicken and cool.

Dice chicken and place in a large bowl, along with the lettuce and mandarin oranges. Toss with the ginger dressing. Spread ½ cup of chicken salad on each wrap.

SERVES 4: 1 WRAP PER PERSON
NUTRITION INFORMATION (PER SERVING): CALORIES: 240 FAT: 2 G
PROTEIN: 27 G

Not Your Grandma's Chicken Salad Pita

4 4-ounce boneless, skinless chicken breasts
2 stalks diced celery
2 small Granny Smith apples, peeled, cored, and diced
½ cup raisins

The Sierras
Solution Recipes:
Decadent-Tasting
Favorites Your Whole
Family Will Love

——

255

½ cup fat-free mayonnaise
2 tablespoons fresh-squeezed lemon juice
2 tablespoons Old Bay Seasoning
Black pepper to taste
4 fat-free pitas

Place chicken in a 4-quart stockpot, add water to cover, and bring to a boil. Lower heat to a simmer and cook until chicken is done, about 18 to 20 minutes. Drain chicken and cool.

Dice chicken and place in a large bowl along with the celery, apple, and raisins. Add mayonnaise, lemon juice, Old Bay Seasoning, and black pepper. Mix thoroughly.

Stuff each pita with 4 ounces of chicken salad. Serve immediately.

SERVES 4: 1 4-OUNCE PITA PER PERSON
NUTRITION INFORMATION (PER SERVING): CALORIES: 189 FAT: 2.6 G
PROTEIN: 34 G

Quiche Florentine

Nonfat cooking spray
1 medium red onion, diced
10 ounces (1 box) frozen chopped spinach, thawed
¼ cup plain breadcrumbs
2 cups fat-free milk
8 egg whites or 1 cup Egg Beaters
¼ cup fat-free Parmesan
1 teaspoon garlic salt
1 teaspoon Old Bay Seasoning
½ teaspoon black pepper

The

Sierras

Solution

Eating

Plan

———

256

Preheat oven to 350°F.

Spray a medium skillet with nonfat cooking spray and heat over medium heat. Sauté the onion for 5 to 6 minutes until almost tender.

Squeeze excess water from thawed spinach until nearly dry. Add spinach to skillet, cooking until all moisture is evaporated.

Add breadcrumbs to mixture, stir, and place in a 9 × 2-inch deep-dish pie pan sprayed with nonfat cooking spray.

Combine all other ingredients in a mixing bowl. Pour over vegetables in deep-dish pie pan.

Bake for 40 to 45 minutes, until firm in center. Allow to stand for 5 to 8 minutes before serving.

SERVES 6: 1 SLICE PER PERSON
NUTRITION INFORMATION (PER SERVING): CALORIES: 111 FAT: 2 G
PROTEIN: 12 G

Sharon's Chicken Taco Salad

6 5-ounce boneless, skinless chicken breasts
Salt and pepper to taste
1½ cups shredded lettuce
1½ cups diced tomatoes
¼ cup chopped scallions
1¼ cups shredded fat-free cheddar cheese
½ cup chopped fresh cilantro
6 ounces fat-free chili lime chips
Salsa or fat-free sour cream, for serving

Heat a grill over medium high heat. Season the chicken with salt and pepper. Grill each breast for 4 minutes per side, or until cooked through. Set aside. (Chicken may also be broiled or purchased precooked.)

In a large bowl, combine lettuce, tomatoes, scallions, cheese, and cilantro. Toss together well.

Divide vegetable mixture evenly into six bowls. Slice chicken into strips and place 5 ounces on top of each bowl of lettuce. Garnish with tortilla chips and serve with salsa or fat-free sour cream, if desired.

SERVES 6: 5 OUNCES CHICKEN STRIPS, SALAD MIX, AND 1 OUNCE CHIPS
PER PERSON
NUTRITION INFORMATION (PER SERVING): CALORIES: 306 FAT: 3.7 G
PROTEIN: 43 G

The Sierras
Solution Recipes:
Decadent-Tasting
Favorites Your Whole
Family Will Love

—

Who Are You Calling Chicken? Enchiladas

Nonfat cooking spray
1 cup diced onion
1½ cups shredded cooked chicken breast
1 cup shredded fat-free cheddar cheese
1 cup jarred picante sauce
3 ounces fat-free cream cheese
1 teaspoon cumin
8 fat-free flour tortillas
1½ cups jarred green taco sauce

Preheat oven to 350°F.

Spray a large skillet with nonfat cooking spray and heat over medium heat.

Add onion and sauté until tender.

Add chicken, ½ cup cheddar cheese, picante sauce, cream cheese, and cumin. Cook until cheese melts, 2 to 3 minutes.

Spoon about ⅓ cup of the chicken mixture down the center of each tortilla, and roll up.

Spray a 13 × 9-inch baking dish with nonfat cooking spray. Place the enchiladas in the prepared dish, drizzle with taco sauce, and sprinkle with the remaining ½ cup of cheddar cheese. Cover and bake until cheese melts, about 15 minutes.

Serve immediately with salsa or fat-free sour cream, if desired.

SERVES 8: 1 ENCHILADA PER PERSON
NUTRITION INFORMATION (PER SERVING): CALORIES: 152 FAT: 1.5 G
PROTEIN: 14 G

The
Sierras
Solution
Eating
Plan

—

258

Dinner

Acorn Squash Ravioli

1 medium acorn squash
Nonfat cooking spray
1 cup fat-free chicken broth
1 tablespoon minced garlic
½ cup diced yellow onion
½ cup fat-free ricotta
⅓ cup minced fresh basil
Salt and pepper to taste
50-count package of wonton wrappers
3 tablespoons cornstarch
⅓ cup grated fat-free Parmesan
¼ cup diced tomato
2 tablespoons chopped flat-leaf parsley

Preheat oven to 425°F.

Cut the acorn squash in half and remove the seeds. Spray a jelly-roll pan with nonfat cooking spray and place the squash on the pan, cut side down. Add ½ inch of water and bake, uncovered, until tender, 30 to 40 minutes. Remove from heat and let it cool.

In medium skillet, heat ¼ cup chicken broth over medium high heat and sauté the garlic and onion until the onion is translucent. Remove from heat, place in a large bowl, and let it cool.

Scoop out the squash and place it in the large bowl with the chicken broth mixture. Add ricotta, basil, salt, and pepper. Mash to a coarse paste using two large forks or a potato masher.

Bring a large pot of water to boil. To create the ravioli, place a wonton wrapper on a lightly floured surface. Place a spoonful of filling, about the diameter of a 50-cent piece and about ¼ inch thick, onto the center of the wrapper. Mix the cornstarch with 3 tablespoons of cold water, and lightly wet the edges of the wonton with the cornstarch mixture. Lay a second wrapper

The Sierras Solution Recipes: Decadent-Tasting Favorites Your Whole Family Will Love

—

over the filling and press the edges onto the bottom piece, removing any trapped air. Trim edges with a ravioli cutter, a pizza cutter, or a sharp knife.

Carefully place filled ravioli in the pot of boiling water, one at a time, while stirring gently. Cook for 5 to 6 minutes. Heat the remaining ¾ cup of chicken broth in a small saucepan.

Remove the cooked ravioli with slotted spoon and place in a shallow bowl. Drizzle with the warmed chicken broth and garnish with Parmesan, tomato, and parsley. Serve immediately.

SERVES 6: 4 RAVIOLI PER PERSON
NUTRITION INFORMATION (PER SERVING): CALORIES: 315 FAT: 2 G
PROTEIN: 16 G

All Gobbled Up Roasted Turkey Breast

½ cup chopped fresh herbs, such as thyme, rosemary, and
   basil
2 tablespoons seasoning salt (preferably Lawry's)
2 tablespoons garlic salt
3-pound fresh turkey breast, boneless, skin on
Nonfat cooking spray
2 tablespoons paprika

Preheat oven to 375°F.

Place the chopped fresh herbs in a small bowl. Add the seasoning salt and garlic salt, and stir.

Rinse turkey and pat dry. Stuff herb mix under the skin of the turkey.

Spray the outside of turkey with nonfat cooking spray and top with paprika and more seasoning salt if desired.

Roast turkey for 1 hour and 45 minutes, or until its internal temperature reaches 165°, or until juices run clear.

SERVES 12: 4 OUNCES PER PERSON
NUTRITION INFORMATION (PER SERVING): CALORIES: 151 FAT: 1 G
PROTEIN: 34 G

The
Sierras
Solution
Eating
Plan

—

260

All Juiced Up Pork Tenderloin

¼ cup jarred plum sauce
¼ cup jarred hoisin sauce
1 teaspoon minced garlic
1 teaspoon minced fresh ginger
Salt and pepper to taste
12-ounce pork tenderloin

Preheat oven to 450°F. Set oven rack to middle of oven.

Place the plum sauce, hoisin sauce, garlic, and ginger in a small bowl.

Put the tenderloin on a foil-lined jelly-roll pan. Tuck the thin end of the tenderloin under to prevent it from overcooking and drying out.

Season the tenderloin with salt and pepper and rub in. Coat the tenderloin liberally with the sauce mixture, covering it entirely.

Roast, uncovered, until the tenderloin is done, about 20 to 25 minutes.

Remove from the oven and let stand about 5 minutes before slicing and serving. This helps keep the juices in and will ensure a moist tenderloin.

SERVES 3: 4 OUNCES PER PERSON
NUTRITION INFORMATION (PER SERVING): CALORIES: 221 FAT: 5 G
PROTEIN: 26 G

Apple of My Eye Pork Stir-Fry

2 tablespoons all-fruit apricot jam
2 tablespoons soy sauce
½ teaspoon cornstarch
Nonfat cooking spray
1 tablespoon minced garlic
1 tablespoon minced fresh ginger
12-ounce pork tenderloin, cut into thin strips
1 cup chopped red bell pepper
1 cup chopped yellow bell pepper
1 cup snow peas
8 ounces water chestnuts, rinsed, drained, and sliced

The Sierras
Solution Recipes:
Decadent-Tasting
Favorites Your Whole
Family Will Love

———

2 unpeeled firm Gala or Fuji apples, cut into 1-inch pieces
½ cup thinly sliced scallions
Black pepper

In a small bowl, place the jam, soy sauce, 2 tablespoons cold water, and cornstarch. Stir and set aside.

Spray a large nonstick skillet with nonfat cooking spray and heat over medium high heat.

Add garlic and ginger and sauté briefly until you start to smell their aromas. Add the pork and stir-fry until the pork is browned and just cooked through, about 3 to 5 minutes. Transfer the pork to a bowl and cover.

Spray the skillet again with nonfat cooking spray. Stir-fry the peppers, snow peas, water chestnuts, and apples until peppers are crisp-tender, about 4 to 5 minutes.

Add the pork back to the skillet, along with the scallions. Stir-fry for 30 seconds.

Stir the jam mixture to recombine, then blend into the stir-fry, stirring constantly. The sauce will thicken fast, in about 30 seconds to 1 minute. Season with the pepper.

Serve immediately over brown rice or whole-wheat pasta, if desired.

SERVES 4: 6 OUNCES PER PERSON
NUTRITION INFORMATION (PER SERVING): CALORIES: 351 FAT: 3 G
PROTEIN: 17 G

Balsamic Baked Chicken

The
Sierras
Solution
Eating
Plan
———
262

Nonfat cooking spray
6 4-ounce boneless, skinless chicken breasts
½ teaspoon black pepper
3 garlic cloves, minced
4½ teaspoons tomato paste
½ cup fat-free chicken broth
⅔ cup balsamic vinegar
¼ cup thinly sliced scallions, green parts only
1 tablespoon honey

Spray a large skillet with nonfat cooking spray and heat over medium high heat.

Season the chicken with pepper, add to skillet, and cook, turning and browning all sides for about 10 minutes. Remove the chicken from the pan and set aside.

Add the garlic to the pan and sauté over medium heat for 2 minutes.

Stir in the tomato paste and slowly add the chicken broth, scraping any bits clinging to the bottom of the pan. Increase the heat to medium high. Stir in the vinegar, scallions, and honey. Boil rapidly for 3 minutes to reduce liquid to 1 cup.

Return the chicken to the pan and reduce the heat to medium. Cook, turning frequently, for about 30 minutes, or until liquid thickens and becomes a dark brown glaze and chicken is done. Serve immediately.

Serves 6: 1 4-ounce chicken breast per person
Nutrition Information (per serving): Calories: 173 Fat: 1.5 g
Protein: 26 g

Cheesy Chicken And Mushroom Casserole

Nonfat cooking spray
4 4-ounce boneless, skinless chicken breasts
¼ teaspoon black pepper
1 teaspoon chili powder
1 cup sliced white button mushrooms
1 cup shredded fat-free cheddar cheese
½ cup fat-free milk
2 cups cubed bread, such as French baguette

Preheat the oven to 350°F.

Spray a 13 × 9-inch baking dish with nonfat cooking spray. Place chicken in the dish and sprinkle with pepper and chili powder.

Top with mushrooms, cheese, and milk. Last, scatter the bread cubes over the top and bake for 40 minutes.

Let casserole cool slightly, then serve immediately.

The Sierras
Solution Recipes:
Decadent-Tasting
Favorites Your Whole
Family Will Love

———

Serves 4: 1 chicken breast per person
Nutrition Information (per serving): Calories: 240 Fat: 1.5 g
Protein: 14 g

Chicken Piccata

4 4-ounce boneless, skinless chicken breasts
3 tablespoons all-purpose flour
Salt and pepper to taste
½ cup fat-free chicken broth
1 tablespoon fresh-squeezed lemon juice
2 tablespoons capers, drained
Nonfat cooking spray

Place each chicken breast between two sheets of plastic wrap or in a large ziplock bag. Pound until meat is about ¼ inch thick.

Place 2 tablespoons of the flour, salt, and pepper on a large plate, and mix. Coat each chicken piece lightly in the flour mixture on both sides.

In small bowl, add the chicken broth, lemon juice, capers, and the last tablespoon of flour. Mix thoroughly, then set aside.

Spray a large skillet with nonfat cooking spray and heat over medium high heat. Add the chicken and cook for 2 to 4 minutes, turning each piece over after a minute or two. If your pan will not accommodate all pieces at once, spray the pan between batches to prevent sticking. The chicken is done when its juices run clear.

Remove chicken from the pan. Give the broth mixture a quick stir, then add it to the pan. Bring to a boil, stirring constantly, until the mixture thickens. Pour the sauce over the chicken and serve immediately.

Serves 4: 4 ounces per person
Nutrition Information (per serving): Calories: 130 Fat: 1.5 g
Protein: 22 g

The
Sierras
Solution
Eating
Plan

———

264

Chicken Marsala

¼ cup all-purpose flour
Salt and pepper to taste
4 4-ounce boneless, skinless chicken breasts
Nonfat cooking spray
½ cup Marsala wine
Juice of ½ lemon
½ cup fat-free chicken broth
½ cup sliced mushrooms (any type)
1 tablespoon chopped fresh flat-leaf parsley

Mix together the flour, salt, and pepper. Coat chicken with the seasoned flour.

Spray a large skillet with nonfat cooking spray and heat over medium high heat.

Add chicken to the skillet and cook for 8 to 12 minutes. The chicken is done when its juices run clear. Remove the chicken from the skillet and set aside, covered, to keep warm.

Add wine to the skillet and stir until heated. Add lemon juice, chicken broth, and mushrooms. Stir, lower the heat, and cook for about 10 minutes over low heat until the sauce is partially reduced. Add parsley and stir.

Pour the sauce over the chicken and serve immediately.

SERVES 4: 4 OUNCES PER PERSON
NUTRITIONAL INFORMATION (PER SERVING): CALORIES: 198 FAT: 1.5 G
PROTEIN: 33 G

Eat Your Spinach Manicotti

10 ounces frozen chopped spinach
Nonfat cooking spray
2 tablespoons minced garlic
⅔ cup diced onion
15 ounces fat-free ricotta
½ cup fat-free Parmesan

The Sierras
Solution Recipes:
Decadent-Tasting
Favorites Your Whole
Family Will Love

———

265

2 egg whites
¼ teaspoon crushed red pepper
1 tablespoon Splenda sugar
8 manicotti shells
2 cups jarred fat-free spaghetti sauce
Salt and pepper to taste

Preheat the oven to 375°F.

Cook the spinach according to the package directions. Drain well, then place spinach between two paper towels or dish towels and squeeze to remove excess moisture. Set aside.

Spray a medium saucepan with nonfat cooking spray and heat over medium heat. Add the garlic and sauté until you smell the aroma of the garlic. Add the onion and sauté until tender, about 8 minutes. Remove from heat, transfer to a bowl, and let cool.

Add spinach, ricotta, ¼ cup of Parmesan, egg whites, red pepper, and sugar to the bowl. Stir well.

Cook manicotti shells according to package directions, omitting salt and oil, and drain well. Stuff spinach mixture evenly into the cooked shells.

Using a 9 × 13-inch pan, spread ½ cup of the spaghetti sauce over the bottom, covering the entire surface. Place filled shells over the sauce, then pour remaining spaghetti sauce over the shells.

Cover with foil or a lid and bake for 30 minutes, until thoroughly heated. Sprinkle the remaining ¼ cup of Parmesan over the top. Serve immediately.

SERVERS 4: 2 SHELLS PER PERSON
NUTRITION INFORMATION (PER SERVING): CALORIES: 325 FAT: 0.5 G
PROTEIN: 27 G

The

Sierras

Solution

Eating

Plan

——

266

Five-Alarm Roasted Chicken

1 clove garlic, minced
1 6-ounce can of chopped green chilies
2 tablespoons cumin
2 tablespoons cayenne pepper
2 tablespoons chili powder

¼ cup chopped cilantro

4 8-ounce chicken breasts with rib bones and skin (skin will be removed after cooking)

Nonfat cooking spray

Seasoning salt (preferably Lawry's) to taste

Black pepper to taste

Preheat the oven to 400°F.

Place the garlic, chilies, cumin, cayenne, chili powder, cilantro, seasoning salt, and pepper in a small bowl, and stir to mix. Divide into four equal amounts.

Rinse the chicken and pat it dry. Make a pocket under the skin of the chicken breast by poking your finger through the membrane. Work your finger under the skin all the way around the breast without poking through the other side.

Rub the seasoning mixture under the skin, covering the entire breast. Repeat with the remaining chicken breasts.

Spray the chicken skin with nonfat cooking spray, then season skin of breast with the seasoning salt and pepper.

Place the chicken in a 9 × 13-inch casserole dish and put in the oven. Roast for 18 to 25 minutes, until the internal temperature of the chicken reaches 165°F, or until juices run clear.

SERVES 4: 4 OUNCES EACH WITHOUT THE BONE OR SKIN

NUTRITION INFORMATION (PER SERVING): CALORIES: 158 FAT: 3 G

PROTEIN: 27 G

Fresno Beef Stir-Fry

12 ounces eye of round or tip roast

Nonfat cooking spray

1 tablespoon minced garlic

¼ cup soy sauce

2 tablespoons Splenda brown sugar

½ cup fresh snow peas or sugar snap peas

½ cup sliced onion

1 cup chopped bok choy

The Sierras
Solution Recipes:
Decadent-Tasting
Favorites Your Whole
Family Will Love

—

1 tablespoon cornstarch
Salt and pepper to taste

Place the beef in the freezer for 10 to 15 minutes—partially frozen meat is easier to slice. Slice the beef into thin strips about ⅛ inch wide and 3 inches long.

Spray a wok or a large skillet with nonfat cooking spray and heat on high heat. Sauté the garlic briefly, then add beef strips and stir-fry, turning pieces constantly until beef is no longer red, about 3 to 4 minutes. Remove the beef and set it aside.

Put the soy sauce, brown sugar, and ¼ cup of water together in a cup, mix, and then add to the wok. Add the vegetables and cook over high heat until they are tender-crisp, 3 to 4 minutes.

Put the cornstarch and ¼ cup cold water in a bowl and stir until smooth. Push the vegetables aside and add the cornstarch mixture to the wok, stirring constantly. Cook until thickened.

Add beef back to the wok and coat both beef and vegetables with sauce. Serve immediately.

SERVES 4: 4 OUNCES PER PERSON
NUTRITION INFORMATION (PER SERVING): CALORIES: 226 FAT: 5 G
PROTEIN 31 G

Happy as a Clam Pasta

2 pounds fresh whole littleneck clams
¼ cup cooking sherry
Nonfat cooking spray
1 tablespoon minced garlic
8 ounces dried angel-hair pasta
2 cups chopped fresh tomatoes (or canned)
½ cup chopped flat-leaf parsley
Salt and pepper to taste

The
Sierras
Solution
Eating
Plan
—
268

Scrub the clams well and place them in a large pot. Pour the sherry over the clams, cover the pot, and heat over high heat until clams just open, about 4 to 6 minutes. Remove from the heat and set aside, discarding any clams that have not opened.

In a new large pot, bring a gallon of salted water to a boil. Meanwhile, remove the clams from the first large pot and reserve the clam liquid.

Spray a large skillet with nonfat cooking spray and heat over medium high heat. Add the garlic, sauté it for 2 minutes, and then add the reserved clam juice. Reduce the liquid by half over medium high heat.

Add the angel-hair pasta to the boiling water and cook according to the package directions, stirring frequently.

Add the tomatoes to the clam liquid and simmer for 8 to 10 minutes. Add the chopped parsley, salt, and pepper and continue to simmer 1 additional minute. Stir.

Drain the pasta and transfer to a large shallow bowl. Toss with the sauce and arrange the clams on top. Serve immediately.

SERVES 6: 6 OUNCES PER PERSON
NUTRITION INFORMATION (PER SERVING): CALORIES: 301 FAT: 3 G
PROTEIN: 34 G

Heavenly Basil Pasta

Nonfat cooking spray
2 tablespoons minced fresh garlic
2 tablespoons minced shallots
6 tomatoes, chopped
Salt and pepper to taste
2 tablespoons chopped basil
12 ounces dried angel-hair pasta
2 tablespoons grated fat-free Parmesan or romano

In a large stockpot bring a gallon of salted water to a boil.

Spray a medium skillet with nonfat cooking spray and heat over medium high heat. Add the garlic and shallots to the pan and sauté just until the shallots start to turn translucent and you can smell the garlic. Add tomatoes, salt, and pepper and let simmer for 15 minutes.

Add the basil to the sauce and mix well. Let simmer for another 2 minutes.

The Sierras
Solution Recipes:
Decadent-Tasting
Favorites Your Whole
Family Will Love

269

Add the pasta to the boiling water and cook according to the package directions, stirring frequently. Drain the pasta and transfer to a large shallow bowl. Toss with the sauce and serve immediately, topping each serving with 1½ teaspoons of grated cheese.

SERVES 6: 1 CUP PER PERSON
NUTRITION INFORMATION (PER SERVING): CALORIES: 238 FAT: 2 G
PROTEIN: 17 G

Home on the Range Buffaloaf

1½ pounds ground buffalo (buy the leanest, 3% fat)
¼ cup egg whites or Egg Beaters
1 cup fat-free milk
¾ cup fat-free breadcrumbs
1 envelope dry onion soup mix
2 tablespoons ketchup
Salt and pepper to taste
Nonfat cooking spray

Preheat the oven to 350°F.

Combine all of the ingredients (except the nonfat cooking spray) in a medium bowl, mixing well.

Spray a loaf pan with the nonfat cooking spray, press the buffaloaf into the pan, and place in the oven. Bake for 1 hour.

Spoon ketchup down the center of the loaf and return it to the oven to cook an additional 12 to 15 minutes. Serve immediately.

SERVES 6: 4 OUNCES PER PERSON
NUTRITION INFORMATION (PER SERVING): CALORIES: 196 FAT: 2.5 G
PROTEIN: 32 G

The
Sierras
Solution
Eating
Plan
—
270

Mango-licious Barbecued Shrimp

1 large mango, peeled, pitted, and coarsely chopped
1 jalapeño pepper, seeded
1 clove garlic, chopped
¼ cup fresh-squeezed lime or lemon juice
1 teaspoon honey
2 tablespoons chopped fresh cilantro
Salt and pepper to taste
1 pound (12–14 count) shrimp, peeled and deveined
Nonfat cooking spray

In a food processor filled with the blade attachment, place the mango, jalapeño, and garlic and purée. Add the lime juice, honey, and cilantro. Blend. Season with salt and pepper. Depending on how hot you want your sauce, add anywhere from half to all of the jalapeño.

Preheat the grill to medium high.

Place the shrimp in a bowl, along with 2 tablespoons of the mango sauce and additional salt and pepper. Thread the shrimp on metal skewers.

Spray the grill with nonfat cooking spray and grill the shrimp on one side for 2 to 3 minutes, then turn and grill for another 2 to 3 minutes. Serve immediately—perhaps over a bed of baby greens or over pasta or rice, drizzling with the remaining mango sauce.

SERVES 4: 4 SHRIMP PER PERSON
NUTRITION INFORMATION (PER SERVING): CALORIES: 160 FAT: 2 G
PROTEIN: 26 G

My Big Fat Greek Chicken

¼ cup light soy sauce
2 tablespoons cooking sherry
2 garlic cloves, minced
3 tablespoons fresh-squeezed lime juice
1 teaspoon minced fresh ginger
¼ teaspoon curry powder

The Sierras
Solution Recipes:
Decadent-Tasting
Favorites Your Whole
Family Will Love

———

271

¼ teaspoon dried oregano, crumbled
¼ teaspoon dried thyme, crumbled
4 4-ounce skinless boneless chicken breasts
1 small onion, sliced thin

In a large glass casserole dish, stir together ¼ cup water, soy sauce, sherry, garlic, lime juice, ginger, curry powder, oregano, and thyme.

Add chicken and marinate, covered and chilled, turning occasionally, for at least 1 hour and up to 24 hours.

Remove the chicken from marinade and pat dry with a paper towel. Reserve marinade.

Spray a large skillet with nonfat cooking spray and heat over medium high heat. Add the chicken to the pan and brown each side, about 1 minute per side. Transfer the chicken to a plate.

Deglaze the skillet with 2 tablespoons of water, using a wooden spoon to scrape up the brown bits on the bottom of the pan. Cook for 1 minute.

Add the onion and cook until soft and tender, 8 to 10 minutes.

Add the chicken, the reserved marinade, and ¼ cup of water to the pan. Simmer, covered, for the next 10 minutes or until chicken is cooked through, basting frequently.

Serve warm.

SERVES 4: 4 OUNCES PER PERSON
NUTRITION INFORMATION (PER SERVING): CALORIES: 159 FAT: 2 G
PROTEIN: 29 G

No Bones About It Garlic Chicken

The
Sierras
Solution
Eating
Plan
———
272

4 8-ounce chicken breasts, with rib bones and skin (skin
*   will be removed after cooking)*
1 clove garlic, minced
Seasoning salt (preferably Lawry's), to taste
Black pepper to taste
Nonfat cooking spray

Preheat oven to 400°F.

Rinse the chicken and pat it dry. Make a pocket under the skin by poking your finger through the membrane. Work your finger under the skin all the way around the breast without poking through the other side. Lift the skin and add the garlic, seasoning salt, and pepper, rubbing it around to cover the entire breast.

Spray the skin of the chicken with nonfat cooking spray, then sprinkle more seasoning salt and pepper on top.

Roast the chicken for 18 to 25 minutes, until the internal temperature of the chicken reaches 165°F, or until juices run clear.

Remember: Cooking with the skin on will not impart fat into the chicken meat. Just don't forget to remove the skin before eating because that is where most of the fat is.

SERVES 4: 4 OUNCES PER PERSON (WITHOUT THE BONE)
NUTRITION INFORMATION (PER SERVING, MEAT ONLY, NO SKIN):
CALORIES: 142 FAT: 3 G PROTEIN: 27 G
NUTRITION INFORMATION (PER SERVING, MEAT WITH SKIN):
CALORIES: 193 FAT: 8 G PROTEIN: 29 G

Makes a difference removing the skin, doesn't it?

Orange You Glad It's Scallops?

Nonfat cooking spray
1 tablespoon minced garlic
1 pound sea or bay scallops
Salt and pepper to taste
¾ cup orange juice
1 teaspoon orange zest
2 teaspoons cornstarch

Spray a medium skillet with nonfat cooking spray and heat over medium high heat.

Add garlic and sauté briefly, until you can smell the garlic. Season the scallops with salt and pepper, then add to the skillet and sauté until slightly

The Sierras
Solution Recipes:
Decadent-Tasting
Favorites Your Whole
Family Will Love
—

brown, about 4 minutes, turning scallops over after the first 2 minutes. Remove and cover to keep warm.

Deglaze the skillet with orange juice, add the orange zest, and bring to a boil.

In small bowl, mix ¼ cup cold water and cornstarch, stirring until completely blended.

Add the cornstarch slurry to the boiling juice in the skillet a little at a time, stirring constantly until mixture starts to thicken. You may not need all the slurry to thicken the sauce.

Add the scallops to the sauce and cook until scallops are heated and covered in sauce, 1 to 2 minutes.

Serve immediately over rice or pasta.

SERVES 4: 4 OUNCES PER PERSON
NUTRITION INFORMATION (PER SERVING): CALORIES: 154 FAT: 2 G
PROTEIN: 26 G

Parmesan-Encrusted Tilapia

½ cup egg whites or Egg Beaters
1½ cups panko (Japanese breadcrumbs)
¼ cup grated fat-free Parmesan
2 tablespoons seasoning salt (preferably Lawry's)
1 teaspoon black pepper
4 4-ounce tilapia fillets (see note)
Nonfat cooking spray

Preheat the oven to 375°F.

Add the egg whites to a small bowl and beat lightly.

In separate bowl, add the panko, Parmesan, seasoning salt, and black pepper. Stir to combine.

Dip fish fillets into egg whites and coat thoroughly, then dip into breadcrumb mixture.

Spray a baking sheet with nonfat cooking spray, add the fillets, and bake for 10 to 12 minutes, turning after 5 or 6 minutes, until golden brown. Serve immediately.

The
Sierras
Solution
Eating
Plan
———
274

Note: Tilapia is a medium- to firm-fleshed white fish, mild and sweet.

SERVES 4: 4 OUNCES PER PERSON
NUTRITION INFORMATION (PER SERVING): CALORIES: 235 FAT: 4 G
PROTEIN: 37 G

Pasta with Garlic Shrimp and Olives

2 tablespoons cooking sherry
1 tablespoon orange juice
¼ cup jarred pimento, diced
5 black California olives
1 tablespoon chopped fresh flat-leaf parsley
2 cloves garlic, minced
1 teaspoon capers, drained
1 teaspoon tomato paste
Salt and pepper to taste
6 ounces shrimp, peeled and deveined
3 ounces dried pasta, such as angel hair or fusilli

In a large pot, bring a gallon of salted water to boil.

Combine the sherry, orange juice, pimento, olives, parsley, garlic, capers, tomato paste, salt, and pepper in a medium skillet. Bring to a boil and then lower heat to a simmer.

Add the shrimp and cook 2 to 4 minutes or until shrimp turn pink. Remove from heat.

Meanwhile, add the pasta to the boiling water and cook according to the package directions, stirring frequently. Drain the pasta, add to the skillet, and toss, blending all ingredients. Serve immediately.

SERVES 2: 9 OUNCES PER PERSON
NUTRITION INFORMATION (PER SERVING): CALORIES: 290 FAT: 2.5 G
PROTEIN 23 G

The Sierras
Solution Recipes:
Decadent-Tasting
Favorites Your Whole
Family Will Love

—

Pork Chops au Poivre

2 tablespoons paprika
1 tablespoon garlic salt
2 teaspoons coarsely ground black pepper
3 tablespoons Worcestershire sauce
2 tablespoons soy sauce
2 tablespoons rice wine vinegar
4 4-ounce center-cut pork loin chops

Heat a grill to medium high heat or preheat the broiler.

Mix all ingredients except the pork chops in a small bowl.

Rub both sides of the pork chops with the mixture, and refrigerate for at least 20 minutes and up to 2 hours.

Grill or broil for about 7 to 9 minutes, or until the pork is done (thermometer reads 160°F).

SERVES 4: 4 OUNCES PER PERSON
NUTRITION INFORMATION (PER SERVING): CALORIES: 167 FAT: 4 G
PROTEIN: 26 G

Reedley's Best Pizza

3 red or yellow bell peppers
Nonfat cooking spray
1 red onion, sliced into thin strips
1 loaf frozen dough for whole-wheat or French bread,
  thawed
½ cup fat-free ricotta
1 large tomato, chopped
½ cup grated fat-free mozzarella
¼ cup grated fat-free Parmesan
2 tablespoons chopped basil
Salt and pepper to taste

The
Sierras
Solution
Eating
Plan

276

Preheat the oven to 425°F.

Cut the peppers in half and remove the seeds and white membranes.

Line a baking sheet with foil and spray the foil with nonfat cooking spray. Place the peppers, cut side down, along with the onion on the baking sheet. Spray the onion lightly with nonfat cooking spray. Place the baking sheet in oven and bake for 10 minutes. Remove the onion and set aside, leaving the peppers on the baking sheet.

Bake peppers for an additional 10 or 15 minutes, until skin is bubbly and browned. Wrap peppers in the foil and let stand until cool enough to handle. Gently rub off the skins of the peppers, and then cut them into 1-inch strips.

Meanwhile, spray a rectangular baking sheet with nonfat cooking spray. Remove the thawed dough from the package and roll it out to fit the sheet. If you like thin-crust pizza, you can divide the dough in half and roll out enough dough for two 12-inch rectangular cookie sheets.

Pat the dough onto the cookie sheet, building up the edges slightly. Prick the crust with a fork. Do not let the dough rise. Place the dough in the oven and bake for about 10 minutes, until lightly browned. Remove from oven and let cool.

Add the ricotta to a small bowl and season with salt and pepper. Using a plastic spatula, spread the ricotta on the dough, covering the entire surface. Distribute the vegetables evenly onto the dough. Top with the mozzarella and basil, and finish by adding the Parmesan evenly over the entire top surface of the pizza.

Cook pizza 12 to 15 minutes, until cheese has completely melted. Serves immediately.

SERVES 8: 1 SLICE PER PERSON

NUTRITION INFORMATION (PER SERVING): CALORIES: 238 FAT: 3 G
PROTEIN: 15 G

Roasted Salmon Fillet

Nonfat cooking spray
1 clove garlic, minced

The Sierras
Solution Recipes:
Decadent-Tasting
Favorites Your Whole
Family Will Love

—

277

8 sprigs fresh tarragon, thyme, or dill
4 4-ounce low-fat salmon fillets, such as pink (humpback)
  or chum

Preheat the oven to 375°F.

Lightly spray a large, oven-safe sauté pan with nonfat cooking spray. Heat the pan on medium high heat.

Add the garlic and sauté briefly. Once you can smell the garlic, add the herbs and heat until you can smell their fragrance.

Add the salmon fillets and brown one side for 2 to 3 minutes. Once one side is browned, turn the fillet over in the pan and place the pan in the oven. Cook salmon for 6 to 8 minutes until medium in temperature, slightly dark pink on the inside. Serve immediately over a bed of jasmine rice or a bed of baby mixed greens.

Salmon can be high in fat, so be sure to pick one of the low-fat varieties listed in the ingredients.

SERVES 4: 4 OUNCES PER PERSON
NUTRITION INFORMATION (PER SERVING): CALORIES: 166 FAT: 5.5 G
PROTEIN: 32 G

Southwestern Chicken Rollatini

4 4-ounce skinless, boneless chicken breasts
½ cup grated fat-free mozzarella
2 jalapeño peppers, minced (seeded if less heat is desired)
¼ cup julienne-sliced red bell pepper
¼ cup chopped fresh cilantro
Nonfat cooking spray

Preheat oven to 375°F.

Place each chicken breast between two sheets of plastic wrap. Pound until meat is about ¼ inch thick. Lay the chicken on a work surface on top of the plastic wrap. Sprinkle 2 tablespoons of mozzarella down the middle of each chicken breast horizontally, then add 1 tablespoon each of the jalapeño, red pepper, and cilantro.

The
Sierras
Solution
Eating
Plan

278

Using the plastic wrap as a support, roll one end of the chicken breast so it just overlaps the stuffing. Tuck the end under and keep rolling. Secure with toothpicks.

Spray a medium skillet with nonfat cooking spray. Brown the chicken 2 to 3 minutes on each side. Arrange chicken rolls in a 9 × 13-inch baking dish. Bake for 30 minutes, until chicken is no longer pink and juices run clear.

SERVES 4: 4 OUNCES PER PERSON
NUTRITION INFORMATION (PER SERVING): CALORIES: 224 FAT: 2 G
PROTEIN: 46 G

Spaghetti Bison Pie

> 4 ounces dried spaghetti
> 1 pound ground buffalo (look for the leanest, 3% fat)
> 1 sweet onion, chopped
> 1 14-ounce can stewed tomatoes, undrained
> 1 15-ounce can tomato sauce
> 1 tablespoon dried oregano
> 1 teaspoon dried thyme
> 1 teaspoon dried basil
> Salt and pepper to taste
> Nonfat cooking spray
> 1 cup fat-free, small-curd cottage cheese
> 1 cup grated fat-free mozzarella
> 3 tablespoons grated Parmesan

Bring a large pot of salted water to boil, add the spaghetti, and cook according to the package directions. Drain and set aside.

Brown the buffalo meat and onion in a large skillet over medium heat for 12 to 15 minutes.

Add tomatoes (and juice from the can), tomato sauce, oregano, thyme, basil, salt, and pepper to the skillet. Simmer for 20 to 25 minutes, uncovered, until it thickens slightly. Set aside.

Preheat the oven to 375°F.

The Sierras
Solution Recipes:
Decadent-Tasting
Favorites Your Whole
Family Will Love

——

Spray a 10-inch glass pie pan with nonfat cooking spray and arrange the spaghetti on the bottom of the pan, creating a crust.

Spread cottage cheese evenly over the spaghetti. Spread meat sauce evenly over the cottage cheese, then top with mozzarella. Sprinkle grated Parmesan over the top of the mozzarella evenly.

Bake in the oven for about 40 minutes, until cheese has turned a golden brown.

SERVES 6: 1 CUP PER PERSON
NUTRITION INFORMATION (PER SERVING): CALORIES: 275 FAT: 3 G
PROTEIN: 33 G

Sweet and Sour Lychee Chicken Stir-Fry

4 4-ounce skinless, boneless chicken breasts
1 8-ounce can lychees, packed in water
1 cup chopped broccoli
1 cup sugar snap peas
1 cup chopped baby bok choy (or regular bok choy)
1 cup sliced yellow onions
Nonfat cooking spray
¼ cup soy sauce
2 tablespoons Splenda brown sugar
1 tablespoon minced fresh ginger
2 tablespoons cornstarch

Cut the chicken breasts into strips approximately ½ inch wide.

Drain the lychees and put into a medium bowl, reserving the liquid separately. Add the vegetables to the bowl and mix.

Spray a wok or large sauté pan with nonfat cooking spray. Add the chicken strips to the wok, then brown and cook the chicken 12 to 15 minutes until juices run clear. Remove from the pan, transfer to a bowl, and cover.

In a separate small bowl, add ¼ cup of the lychee water, soy sauce, brown sugar, and ginger. Mix thoroughly.

Deglaze the wok or sauté pan with the lychee mixture, scraping any bits clinging to the bottom of the pan. Bring to a boil.

The
Sierras
Solution
Eating
Plan
———
280

Add the vegetables and cook until broccoli is fork-tender. Once the broccoli is done, the remaining vegetables will be done as well. Reduce the heat to medium.

In a bowl or cup, add ¼ cup lukewarm water and stir in the cornstarch, mixing thoroughly. Push the vegetables aside in the wok and add the cornstarch mixture slowly to the sauce. Keep stirring until the sauce thickens. You may not need all of the cornstarch mixture.

Add the chicken back to the wok to reheat. Toss the chicken and vegetables to make sure they are completely coated. Serve immediately over rice.

Serves 4: 4 ounces each
Nutrition Information (per serving): Calories: 172.5 Fat: 1.7 g
Protein: 28.3 g

Sweet Potato Couscous

2 medium sweet potatoes
Nonfat cooking spray
2 tablespoons minced garlic
1 teaspoon curry powder
½ teaspoon dried nutmeg
2 red bell peppers, chopped
1 28-ounce can diced or chopped tomatoes (do not drain)
1 teaspoon salt
½ teaspoon crushed red pepper
Black pepper to taste
2 cups uncooked regular couscous

Peel the sweet potatoes and cut into ½-inch cubes.

Spray a Dutch oven (or other large, heavy pot with a close-fitting lid) with nonfat cooking spray. Add garlic, curry powder, nutmeg, and sweet potatoes. Cook over medium heat for about 5 minutes.

Add the peppers, increase the heat to medium high, cover, and cook for 5 minutes. Uncover and cook for 5 minutes more, stirring occasionally.

Increase the heat to high; add tomatoes and juice. Bring to a boil and add salt, crushed red pepper, and black pepper.

The Sierras
Solution Recipes:
Decadent-Tasting
Favorites Your Whole
Family Will Love

———

281

Reduce the heat to low and simmer for about 15 minutes, until sweet potatoes are tender.

Bring three cups of water and ½ teaspoon salt to boil in a small pot. Add couscous, cover, and remove from the heat. Let stand for 5 minutes.

Fluff the couscous with a fork, spoon sweet potato mixture over couscous, and serve immediately.

SERVES 6: 2.5 OUNCES PER PERSON
NUTRITION INFORMATION (PER SERVING): CALORIES: 204 FAT: 1 G
PROTEIN: 7 G

Tuna Patties

*1 12-ounce can light white tuna packed in water, drained
  and finely flaked*
¾ cup fat-free seasoned breadcrumbs
¼ cup minced scallions
2 tablespoons drained and chopped pimentos
Scant ¼ cup egg whites or 3 tablespoons Egg Beaters
½ cup fat-free milk
½ teaspoon lemon zest
1 tablespoon Old Bay Seasoning

In a large bowl, combine tuna, breadcrumbs, scallions, pimentos, egg whites, milk, lemon zest, and Old Bay Seasoning. Mix well and form into 8 patties.

Spray a large skillet with nonfat cooking spray and heat over medium heat. Sauté patties a few at a time until golden brown on both sides, about 3 minutes per side. Serve immediately.

SERVES 4: 2 PATTIES PER PERSON
NUTRITION INFORMATION (PER SERVING): CALORIES: 265 FAT: 1.25 G
PROTEIN: 29 G

The
Sierras
Solution
Eating
Plan

282

Very Veggie Stuffed Bell Peppers

Nonfat cooking spray
1 tablespoon minced garlic
1 red onion, sliced
1 medium zucchini, diced
½ cup sliced white button mushrooms
1 14-ounce can chopped tomatoes, drained
1 tablespoon tomato paste
2 tablespoons chopped fresh basil
Salt and pepper to taste
4 medium-size red bell peppers, cut in half lengthwise and
*   seeded*
¼ cup grated fat-free Parmesan

Preheat oven to 350°F.

Spray a large saucepan with nonfat cooking spray and heat over medium heat.

Add the garlic and sauté briefly until you smell the aroma of the garlic. Add the onion, zucchini, and mushrooms and cook for 3 minutes, stirring occasionally.

Stir in the tomatoes and tomato paste. Increase the heat to high and bring the mixture to a boil, then reduce the heat to low, simmering for 10 to 15 minutes, until the mixture is slightly thickened. Remove from heat and stir in the basil, salt, and pepper.

Fill a medium saucepan with water about halfway and bring to a boil. Blanch the pepper halves for about 3 minutes and then drain.

Place the peppers, cut side up, in a shallow ovenproof dish and fill with the vegetable mixture. Cover with foil or a lid and bake for 20 minutes. After 20 minutes, uncover and sprinkle Parmesan over the peppers. Return to the oven, uncovered, for another 5 to 10 minutes.

SERVES 4: 1 STUFFED PEPPER PER PERSON
NUTRITION INFORMATION (PER SERVING): CALORIES: 165 FAT: 0 G
PROTEIN: 7 G

The Sierras
Solution Recipes:
Decadent-Tasting
Favorites Your Whole
Family Will Love
—

Notes on Recipes

Lunch vs. Dinner

Some of the lunch recipes can be used as dinner entrées, and vice versa. Feel free to indulge your taste buds whenever with any of these items. Enjoy!

Nonfat cooking spray

Even though these sprays say "0 grams of fat per serving," keep in mind that they are still made with oil and that the "0 grams of fat per serving" simply means that the recommended serving size is so small that the grams of fat can be legally rounded down to zero on the label. So use this sparingly, and certainly stop spraying before you form a small pool. Otherwise, you might as well be using oil.

Pasta

Remember that pasta doesn't measure dry the same as cooked. Here is an easy way to remember how much pasta to use the next time you are cooking for more than one:

- 8 ounces of dried pasta will make 4 cups of cooked pasta. That is, 4 servings if each serving is 1 cup.
- 12 ounces of dried pasta will make 6 cups of cooked pasta, and so on.

Buffalo

Buffalo (otherwise known as bison) is an AOS and Wellspring favorite, with about a quarter the fat of beef. We enjoy buffalo in burgers, Sloppy Joes, and the recipes included in this book.

Keep these tips in mind when cooking buffalo:

- Roasting—Set your oven temperature between 250°F and 275°F and use a meat thermometer to check for doneness at 110°F to 120°F.
- Grilling and broiling—After searing the meat, you want to make sure to keep it moist, so low temperatures and slow cooking are the key. Using barbecue sauce or a marinade also helps keep meat moist.

(continued)

■ Remember, if you have a tough piece of buffalo meat, the toughness is more than likely due to the way it was cooked, not the meat itself. The rule of thumb with buffalo is to not overcook. Slow and low is the motto when it comes to cooking this lean and low-fat meat!

FINDING BUFFALO

Although buffalo is widely available in specialty and gourmet food stores, it may be hard to find in your local grocery. So ask the meat department, and be sure to check the fat content. Some buffalo can be higher in fat.

If there is no convenient source near you, you can do what we do at AOS and order online from www.buffalogal.com. If you mention AOS, Buffalo Gal tells us you'll receive the same discount we receive.

The Sierras
Solution Recipes:
Decadent-Tasting
Favorites Your Whole
Family Will Love

285

Side Dishes, Soup, and Salads

Baked Light French Fries

6 large russet potatoes
3 tablespoons garlic salt
3 tablespoons seasoning salt (preferably Lawry's)
2 tablespoons black pepper
Nonfat cooking spray
Salt to taste

Preheat the oven to 425°F.

Peel the potatoes and cut into long strips. Place potatoes in a large bowl and rinse thoroughly with cold water. Drain.

In a separate large bowl, place seasonings and stir to combine. Add potatoes and toss until well coated.

Line a baking sheet with foil and spray foil with nonfat cooking spray. Arrange the potatoes in a single layer on the sheet and bake for 15 to 25 minutes, until easily pierced or until golden brown.

Sprinkle with salt and serve hot.

SERVES 4: 4 OUNCES PER PERSON (ABOUT 12 FRIES)
NUTRITION INFORMATION (PER SERVING): CALORIES: 175 FAT: 0 G
PROTEIN: 2.25 G

Baked Potato Latkes

The
Sierras
Solution
Eating
Plan
—
286

Nonfat cooking spray
2 medium yellow onions, diced
2 pounds russet potatoes
⅓ cup egg whites or Egg Beaters
1 tablespoon all-purpose flour
1 tablespoon seasoning salt (preferably Lawry's)
½ teaspoon black pepper
Applesauce or fat-free sour cream, for serving

Preheat the oven to 400°F.

Spray a medium skillet with nonfat cooking spray and heat over medium heat. Sauté the onions until softened, about 10 minutes. Set aside to cool.

Peel and coarsely grate the potatoes. Squeeze out the excess liquid, transfer potatoes to a large bowl, and add the onions, egg whites, flour, seasoning salt, and pepper. Stir to combine.

Spray a muffin pan with nonfat cooking spray. Evenly distribute the potato mixture among the 12 muffin slots. Bake until firm and brown at edges, about 45 minutes.

Serve hot with applesauce or fat-free sour cream, if desired.

SERVES 4: 2 LATKES PER PERSON

NUTRITION INFORMATION (PER SERVING): CALORIES: 188 FAT: 0 G
PROTEIN: 5 G

Blue-Stuffed Tomatoes

1 pound broccoli florets
Salt and pepper to taste
4 large tomatoes
½ cup instant stuffing mix, herb flavor
½ cup fat-free blue cheese dressing
¼ cup grated fat-free Parmesan

Preheat the oven to 425°F.

In a large microwave-safe bowl, place the broccoli along with two tablespoons of water and the salt and pepper. Microwave for 3 to 6 minutes on the highest setting, keeping in mind that all microwaves vary. Check for tenderness after the first 3 minutes. Set aside to cool.

Wash and dry the tomatoes. Slice off the tops of the tomatoes, scoop out the centers, and leave ¼ inch of shell. Drain. Chop the cooled broccoli into small pieces.

In a medium bowl, add the stuffing mix and broccoli and stir to combine. Add the blue cheese dressing and mix until dressing is completely incorporated.

The Sierras
Solution Recipes:
Decadent-Tasting
Favorites Your Whole
Family Will Love

—

287

Spray a 9 × 13-inch baking dish with nonfat cooking spray and place the tomatoes in the dish. Sprinkle Parmesan evenly over each tomato.
Bake for 15 to 20 minutes, until heated through.

SERVES 4: 1 TOMATO PER PERSON
NUTRITION INFORMATION (PER SERVING): CALORIES: 120 FAT: 2 G
PROTEIN 4 G

Candied Carrots

7 or 8 large carrots (14 to 16)
2 teaspoons minced fresh ginger
½ cup raisins or golden raisins
2 tablespoons Splenda brown sugar
1 tablespoon lemon juice

Peel and slice the carrots diagonally into ½-inch slices.
Pour 2 cups of water into a medium saucepan and bring to a boil. Add carrots, ginger, raisins, brown sugar, and lemon juice. Make sure water covers carrots, adding more if necessary. Reduce heat to medium high and cook the carrots for 12 to 15 minutes, until tender.

SERVES 4: ¼ CUP EACH
NUTRITION INFORMATION (PER SERVING): CALORIES: 124 FAT: 2 G
PROTEIN: 1 G

Cheesy Broccoli Bake

4 cups chopped broccoli
Nonfat cooking spray
½ cup chopped yellow onion
1½ cups egg whites or Egg Beaters
1 cup fat-free milk
1½ cups fat-free cheddar cheese
Salt and pepper to taste

The
Sierras
Solution
Eating
Plan

———

288

Preheat oven to 350°F.

Place the broccoli in a large microwave-safe bowl, and microwave on high until tender, about 3 to 5 minutes. Set aside.

Spray a small sauté pan with nonfat cooking spray and heat over medium heat. Sauté the onion till tender, about 10 minutes. Set aside.

In a large bowl, combine the egg whites, milk, and cheese. Mix well. Stir in the broccoli and onion. Add salt and pepper.

Spray a 1½-quart baking dish with nonfat cooking spray. Pour the mixture into the baking dish. Set this dish into a larger roasting pan and fill the outer dish with about 1 inch of water. This will help keep the temperature even while the dish is cooking and prevent the broccoli from drying out.

Bake for 45 minutes. This dish is done when a knife inserted in the center comes out clean. Let cool for about 10 minutes before serving.

SERVES 6: 1 CUP PER PERSON

NUTRITION INFORMATION (PER SERVING): CALORIES: 92 FAT: 0 G

PROTEIN: 11 G

Creamy Mushroom Soup

Nonfat cooking spray
2 teaspoons crushed garlic
1 cup chopped yellow onion
2½ cups fat-free beef or chicken stock
1 cup diced russet potatoes
1¾ cups white button mushrooms, sliced (or any other
*   variety—for a richer soup, use shiitake or oyster mushrooms)*
⅓ cup cooking sherry or Madeira wine
½ cup fat-free milk
Salt and pepper to taste

Spray a medium saucepan with nonfat cooking spray, heat over medium heat, and sauté garlic and onions until softened, approximately 10 minutes.

Add the stock and potatoes, cover, and simmer for 20 to 25 minutes or until softened. Purée until smooth in a food processor fitted with the blade attachment. Return to saucepan and set aside.

The Sierras
Solution Recipes:
Decadent-Tasting
Favorites Your Whole
Family Will Love

———

Spray a medium skillet with nonfat cooking spray and heat over medium heat. Sauté mushrooms 6 to 8 minutes until softened. Add the cooking sherry, cook for 2 to 3 minutes, and then add to soup. Stir thoroughly.

Warm the milk in the microwave or on the stovetop, add to soup, and stir until combined. Add salt and pepper to taste.

Serve immediately.

SERVES 4: 1 CUP PER PERSON
NUTRITION INFORMATION (PER SERVING): CALORIES: 142 FAT: 0.5 G
PROTEIN: 24.2 G

Curried Cauliflower Bake

⅓ cup fat-free plain yogurt
¼ cup grated fat-free Parmesan
¼ teaspoon cumin
¼ teaspoon turmeric
¼ teaspoon curry powder
¼ cup fat-free breadcrumbs
1 tablespoon curry powder
2 pounds cauliflower, cut into florets
Nonfat cooking spray

Preheat the oven to 375°F.

In a small bowl, combine the yogurt, Parmesan, cumin, turmeric, and ¼ teaspoon curry powder. Set aside.

Combine breadcrumbs with tablespoon of curry powder in a separate small bowl. Set aside.

Microwave cauliflower until just tender, 4 to 6 minutes.

Spray an 8-inch square baking pan with nonfat cooking spray and spread the cauliflower out into the pan. Spoon the yogurt mixture over the cauliflower and toss gently to coat.

Sprinkle the breadcrumbs over all. Bake until the crumbs are crisp and well browned, about 20 minutes. Serve immediately.

The
Sierras
Solution
Eating
Plan

———

290

SERVES 6: ¼ CUP PER PERSON
NUTRITION INFORMATION (PER SERVING): CALORIES: 74 FAT: 1 G
PROTEIN: 4 G

Easiest Rice Pilaf Ever

Nonfat cooking spray
¼ cup diced yellow onion
1 cup white rice
1¾ cups fat-free chicken stock or water
1 bay leaf
Salt and pepper to taste

Spray a medium saucepan with nonfat cooking spray and heat over medium heat. Add onion and sauté until tender, about 2 to 3 minutes. Add rice and cook for about 1 minute, stirring constantly.

Add the chicken stock, bay leaf, salt, and pepper and bring to a boil. Once stock reaches a boil, lower the heat and simmer for about 20 to 25 minutes, until all liquid is absorbed. If rice is undercooked, add ¼ cup more stock, cover, and cook an additional 5 to 7 minutes. Rice should be light and fluffy when done.

Serve immediately.

SERVES 6: ½ CUP PER PERSON
NUTRITION INFORMATION (PER SERVING): CALORIES: 63.3 FAT: 0 G
PROTEIN: 2.5 G

Green Bean Casserole

Nonfat cooking spray
1 medium yellow onion, chopped
1 9-ounce package frozen French-style green beans
1 10-ounce can fat-free cream of mushroom soup
½ cup shredded fat-free cheddar cheese
1 28-ounce can Durkee's French-fried Onions

Preheat the oven to 325°F.

Spray a small skillet with nonfat cooking spray and heat over medium heat. Add the onions and sauté until tender. Add green beans and mushroom soup. Stir, then add cheddar cheese.

The Sierras
Solution Recipes:
Decadent-Tasting
Favorites Your Whole
Family Will Love

—

291

Cook for 20 minutes, until heated through. Garnish with Durkee's onions and cook another 5 minutes.

Serve immediately.

Serves 4: approximately ¼ cup per person
Nutrition Information (per serving): Calories: 65 Fat grams: 0 g
Protein: 2 g

Guiltless Mac and Cheese

Nonfat cooking spray
8 ounces dried elbow macaroni
1 tablespoon all-purpose flour
1 cup fat-free milk
4 ounces shredded fat-free cheddar cheese
2 teaspoons dried mustard
Salt and pepper to taste
1½ cups fat-free, small-curd cottage cheese
3 tablespoons fat-free breadcrumbs
3 tablespoons grated fat-free Parmesan or Romano

Preheat the oven to 375°F.

Spray a 2-quart baking dish with nonfat cooking spray and set aside.

Bring a large pot of salted water to boil and cook the macaroni according to the directions on the package. Drain and set aside.

In a small bowl, whisk together flour and 2 tablespoons of the milk.

Heat the remaining milk in a large saucepan until steaming. Gradually whisk in a little hot milk into the bowl with milk-flour mixture, just enough to warm it up. Next, pour the milk-flour mixture into the pan with hot milk and stir over medium heat for about 1 minute, or until mixture comes to a boil and thickens. Remove from heat and stir in the cheddar, mustard, salt, and black pepper; set aside.

In a food processor fitted with the blade attachment or a blender, purée the cottage cheese until very smooth. Stir it into cheese sauce, then stir in the macaroni. Spoon the mixture into the prepared baking dish.

The
Sierras
Solution
Eating
Plan

——

292

In a small bowl, stir together the breadcrumbs and Parmesan. Sprinkle over the top of the macaroni and cheese.

Bake 40 to 45 minutes, until browned and bubbly. Serve immediately.

SERVES 6: ¼ CUP PER PERSON

NUTRITION INFORMATION (PER SERVING): CALORIES: 260 FAT: 1 G

PROTEIN: 20 G

Herb-Roasted Vegetables

Nonfat cooking spray
2 cups sliced white button mushrooms
4 cups broccoli florets
1 cup sliced carrots
1 medium red onion, thinly sliced
½ cup chopped red pepper
1 cup chopped fresh basil
¼ cup fresh thyme, leaves only
½ cup chopped fresh flat-leaf parsley
3 tablespoons grated fat-free Parmesan
4 cloves garlic, minced
1 tablespoon balsamic or apple cider vinegar
½ cup fat-free chicken stock
Salt and black pepper to taste

Preheat the oven to 425° F.

Spray a 9 × 13-inch baking dish with nonfat spray, then add the vegetables. Stir in the basil, thyme, parsley, Parmesan, garlic, vinegar, and chicken stock. Season with salt and pepper.

Bake for 20 to 25 minutes, stirring frequently, until vegetables are tender.

SERVES 8: ½ CUP PER PERSON

NUTRITION INFORMATION (PER SERVING): CALORIES: 55 FAT: 1 G

PROTEIN: 5 G

The Sierras
Solution Recipes:
Decadent-Tasting
Favorites Your Whole
Family Will Love

———

Italian Vegetable Salad

2 cups chopped plum tomatoes
1 cup chopped yellow bell peppers
1 cup chopped red bell peppers
2 cups chopped English cucumbers
½ cup red onion, sliced thin
¼ cup crumbled fat-free feta
½ cup prepared fat-free Italian dressing
Salt and pepper

In a serving bowl, combine tomatoes, peppers, cucumbers, onion, and feta. Pour the dressing over the salad and toss to coat. Add salt and pepper to taste. Serve immediately.

SERVES 12: ¼ CUP PER PERSON
NUTRITION INFORMATION (PER SERVING): CALORIES: 27.8 FAT: 0 G
PROTEIN: 0.6 G

Joe's Wild, Wild Mushroom Risotto

1½ cups fat-free chicken stock
Nonfat cooking spray
1 teaspoon minced garlic
¼ cup diced yellow onion
¼ cup thinly sliced shiitake mushrooms
¼ cup thinly sliced crimini mushrooms
¼ cup sliced white button mushrooms
½ cup Arborio rice
1 tablespoon chopped fresh thyme
Salt and pepper to taste

Heat the chicken stock in a medium saucepan. Keep warm over very low heat.

Spray a medium saucepan with nonfat cooking spray, add garlic, and

The

Sierras

Solution

Eating

Plan

—

294

cook until you can smell the garlic. Add the onion and sauté 6 to 8 minutes until the onion is translucent. Add shitake and crimini mushrooms and cook until they are soft.

Meanwhile, place the button mushrooms in a small microwave-safe bowl and microwave on high for 1 minute, until soft. Purée in a food processor fitted with the blade attachment. Set aside.

Add rice to saucepan, stirring constantly, then slowly add the chicken stock ½ cup at a time. Keep stirring and make sure risotto has absorbed chicken stock each time before adding next batch of stock. The process will take 15 to 20 minutes. Add puréed mushrooms and thyme, salt, and pepper to risotto mixture. Serve immediately.

SERVES 2: ½ CUP PER PERSON
NUTRITION INFORMATION (PER SERVING): CALORIES: 210 FAT: 2 G
PROTEIN: 6.3 G

Leek and Gold Potato Soup

8 Yukon gold potatoes, peeled and cut into ½-inch pieces
2 large leeks, white and pale green parts only, chopped
1 large yellow onion, chopped
1 quart fat-free, low-sodium chicken broth
Black pepper to taste

Combine potatoes, leeks, onion, broth, and pepper in a large pot and bring to a boil. Reduce the heat and simmer, covered, until vegetables are tender, 22 to 25 minutes. Remove from heat and let cool for 10 minutes.

Transfer the mixture to a blender and purée, working in batches if necessary to prevent overflow. You may also keep a few of the potatoes aside to mash roughly with a fork and add to the purée. This will give the soup a heartier consistency. Serve immediately.

SERVES 4: 1 CUP PER PERSON
NUTRITION INFORMATION (PER SERVING): CALORIES: 141 FAT: 0 G
PROTEIN: 4 G

The Sierras
Solution Recipes:
Decadent-Tasting
Favorites Your Whole
Family Will Love

———

Roasted Candied Acorn Squash

2 acorn squashes
Nonfat cooking spray
¼ cup Splenda brown sugar
1 tablespoon minced fresh ginger
1 tablespoon ground allspice

Preheat oven to 400°F.

Slice the tops and bottoms off the squashes and discard. Using a sharp knife, slice each squash into four rings, creating eight rings in all.

Line a baking sheet with foil, spray with nonfat cooking spray, arrange the squash rings in a single layer on the sheet, and bake for 15 minutes.

In small bowl, combine brown sugar, ginger, and allspice. Sprinkle the mixture evenly over the squash rings. Return rings to oven and cook for another 15 to 20 minutes, or until squash is tender.

SERVES 4: 2 RINGS PER PERSON
NUTRITION INFORMATION (PER SERVING): CALORIES: 49.2 FAT: 0 G
PROTEIN 10.8 G

Roasted Caramelized Onions

2 pounds Vidalia or sweet onions (about 4 large)
Nonfat cooking spray
¼ cup balsamic vinegar
2 tablespoons Splenda brown sugar
2 teaspoons dried thyme
Salt and pepper to taste

Preheat oven to 450°F.

Peel the onions, leaving the roots intact. Cut each onion into 6 wedges.

Spray a 9 × 13-inch baking dish with nonfat cooking spray and add the onion wedges.

Mix vinegar, brown sugar, thyme, salt, and pepper in a small bowl, then pour over onion wedges, tossing to coat evenly. Cover and bake for 25 min-

The
Sierras
Solution
Eating
Plan

296

utes. Remove the cover after 25 minutes and continue baking for an additional 45 minutes, until tender. Serve immediately.

SERVES 6: 4 WEDGES PER PERSON
NUTRITION INFORMATION (PER SERVING): CALORIES: 74 FAT: 0 G
PROTEIN: 1 G

Spinach, Raspberry, and Mandarin Orange Salad

6 cups regular or baby spinach leaves, washed, dried, and
*   torn*
1 cup drained canned mandarin orange slices
½ cup red onion, sliced thin
½ cup thinly sliced crimini or white button mushrooms
½ cup fat-free raspberry dressing
½ cup fresh raspberries
Salt and pepper to taste

In a large serving bowl, combine the spinach, oranges, onion, and mushrooms. Toss together. Pour dressing over salad; toss to coat.

To serve, place 1 cup of salad in bowl or plate and garnish with raspberries. Add salt and pepper to taste.

SERVES 6: 1 CUP PER PERSON
NUTRITION INFORMATION (PER SERVING): CALORIES: 62.5 FAT: 1 G
PROTEIN: 1.4 G

Sweet Potato Kugel

Nonfat cooking spray
1 pound sweet potatoes (about 2 medium)
1 medium russet potato
1 medium carrot, finely grated
½ cup golden raisins

The Sierras
Solution Recipes:
Decadent-Tasting
Favorites Your Whole
Family Will Love

—

297

½ cup egg whites or Egg Beaters
¼ cup orange juice
1 teaspoon ground allspice
Salt and pepper to taste
½ cup breadcrumbs or matzo meal

Preheat the oven to 350°F.

Spray an 8-inch-square baking pan with nonfat cooking spray.

Peel and grate the sweet potatoes into a large bowl. Peel and grate the russet potato into a smaller bowl.

Add russet potato to sweet potatoes small handfuls at a time, squeezing as much of the water out as possible. Add carrot and raisins to potato mixture and mix well.

In a small bowl, whisk together the egg whites, orange juice, allspice, salt, and pepper. Add to potatoes and mix to blend well. Add the breadcrumbs and mix well.

Turn the mixture into the prepared baking pan. Press down firmly with a spatula and smooth the surface. Cover the pan with foil.

Bake for 25 minutes. Remove the foil and continue to bake another 25 minutes, until vegetables are tender. Remove from heat and let cool about 15 minutes.

Cut the kugel into 8 equal rectangles and serve warm.

SERVES 8: ¼ CUP PER PERSON

NUTRITION INFORMATION (PER SERVING): CALORIES: 103 FAT: 0.5 G

PROTEIN: 4 G

The
Sierras
Solution
Eating
Plan

———

298

Sweet and Sour Coleslaw

¾ cup chopped snow peas
3 cups shredded green cabbage
3 cups shredded red cabbage
1 cup sliced yellow peppers
1 cup sliced water chestnuts
2 scallions, chopped

DRESSING

    ¼ cup fat-free mayonnaise
    3 tablespoons Splenda brown sugar
    2 tablespoons rice wine vinegar
    1 tablespoon soy sauce
    1 teaspoon minced fresh ginger
    1 teaspoon minced garlic
    Salt and pepper to taste

Place the snow peas on a microwave-safe dish and microwave on high for 1 to 2 minutes until tender-crisp. Immediately plunge into cold water to stop the cooking. Drain.

Add the snow peas to a large serving bowl with the cabbage, peppers, water chestnuts, and scallions. Mix well.

In small bowl, whisk together the mayonnaise, brown sugar, vinegar, soy sauce, ginger, and garlic. Add salt and pepper to taste. Pour over the salad and toss well.

SERVES 12: ½ CUP PER PERSON
NUTRITION INFORMATION (PER SERVING): CALORIES: 44.8 FAT: 0.2 G
PROTEIN: 0.8 G

Sweet and Tart Carrots and Apples

    3 cups Granny Smith apples, peeled and sliced
    1½ cups baby carrots
    ⅛ teaspoon salt
    ½ teaspoon ground cinnamon
    ⅓ cup dried tart cherries
    ½ cup Splenda brown sugar

Place the apples, carrots, ¾ cup water, and salt in 3-quart saucepan. Cover and cook over medium heat until the water starts to boil. Reduce the heat and simmer for 4 minutes, or until carrots are fork-tender. Drain and keep the carrots and apples in the pan.

Add cinnamon and dried tart cherries along with an additional ¾ cup water to pan and toss gently until combined.

The Sierras
Solution Recipes:
Decadent-Tasting
Favorites Your Whole
Family Will Love

———

Cook over medium heat for 5 to 6 minutes, until the brown sugar dissolves and the apples are glazed.

SERVES 8: ½ CUP PER PERSON
NUTRITION INFORMATION (PER SERVING): CALORIES: 137 FAT: 1.5 G
PROTEIN: 1 G

The
Sierras
Solution
Eating
Plan

—

300

Appendix 1:

The Sierras Solution Shopping Lists

Note: Each weekly shopping list is designed to be all-inclusive, in case you choose to start the plan, for example, with the menus for Week Four instead of Week One. Thus, you may not need to buy all of the nonperishable items listed for each week. Check the quantities of the pantry items you have on hand before restocking.

Week One

BAKING AND SPICES

1 box Old Bay Seasoning
1 can baking powder
1 can nonfat cooking spray
1 can salt
1 jar black pepper
1 jar chili powder
1 jar cumin

1 jar paprika
1 jar seasoning salt, preferably Lawry's
1-pound bag Splenda brown sugar
1-pound box cornstarch
5-pound bag all-purpose flour
5-pound bag whole-wheat flour

BREAD

1 loaf Italian bread
1 package English muffins (6 count)
1 package 10-inch fat-free or low-fat flour tortillas (10 or 12 count)

DAIRY

1 gallon fat-free milk

2 quarts Egg Beaters or 6 dozen eggs (for egg whites)

3 8-ounce packages fat-free shredded cheddar cheese

8 ounces fat-free cream cheese

8 ounces fat-free shredded mozzarella

12-ounce package fat-free American cheese slices

FROZEN

1-pound bag blueberries

MEAT AND FISH

1 pound salmon fillet, lean variety (chum, humpback, or pink)

1 pound tilapia fillets

3 pounds boneless, skinless turkey breast

6½ pounds boneless, skinless chicken breasts

8 8-ounce chicken breasts, bone in, skin on

12-ounce package lean Canadian bacon

12-ounce package lean turkey bacon

12 ounces eye of round or tip roast

OTHER STAPLES AND CONDIMENTS

1 bottle fat-free barbecue sauce

1 can fat-free evaporated milk

1 small jar capers

1 small jar pimentos

2 6-ounce cans light tuna

3 4-ounce cans diced green chilies

8-ounce can grated fat-free or reduced-fat Parmesan

8-ounce jar green taco sauce

8-ounce jar picante sauce

12-ounce can fat-free breadcrumbs

12-ounce can fat-free panko (Japanese breadcrumbs)

15-ounce can mandarin oranges in juice

16-ounce bottle fat-free ginger dressing

16-ounce jar medium salsa

25-ounce jar applesauce, unsweetened

PRODUCE

1 bunch fresh basil
1 bunch fresh cilantro
1 bunch fresh dill
1 bunch fresh rosemary
1 bunch scallions
1 bunch fresh tarragon
1 bunch fresh thyme
1 head bok choy
1 head garlic
1 head romaine lettuce
1 jalapeño pepper

1 lemon
1 medium red onion
2 medium tomatoes
2 medium yellow onions
1 plum tomato
1 red bell pepper
4 ounces snow peas
5-ounce package baby spinach
8-ounce package white button
   mushrooms

Week Two

BAKING AND SPICES

1 bottle vanilla extract
1 box Old Bay Seasoning
1 can baking powder
1 can nonfat cooking spray
1 can salt
1 jar crushed red pepper flakes
1 jar curry powder
1 jar garlic salt
1 jar ground allspice

1 jar ground cinnamon
1 jar ground nutmeg
1-pound bag Splenda brown sugar
1-pound box cornstarch
5-pound bag all-purpose flour
5-pound bag whole-wheat flour
16-ounce bottle light corn syrup
18-ounce can quick-cooking oats

BREAD

1 package pita bread (12 count)
1 loaf Italian bread
1 package English muffins (6 count)
1 package 10-inch fat-free flour tortillas (10 or 12 count)

Dairy

1 gallon fat-free milk

1 package fat-free feta

2 quarts Egg Beaters or 6 dozen
  eggs (for egg whites)

8 ounces shredded fat-free
  cheddar cheese

8 ounces shredded fat-free
  mozzarella

12-ounce package fat-free
  American cheese slices

16 ounces fat-free cream
  cheese

Frozen

1-pound bag blueberries

10-ounce box chopped spinach

12-ounce can orange juice concentrate

Meat and Shellfish

1 pound canned lump crabmeat

1 pound sea scallops

7½ pounds boneless, skinless chicken breasts

12-ounce package lean turkey bacon

18 ounces pork tenderloin

Other Staples and Condiments

1 bottle marsala cooking wine

1 can diced tomatoes

1 jar fat-free mayonnaise

1-pound bag chili lime chips,
  preferably Guiltless Gourmet

1 quart fat-free chicken broth

1 small jar all-fruit apricot jam

1 small jar capers

1 small jar pimentos

6-ounce can capers

6-ounce can light tuna

6-ounce can tomato paste

8-ounce bottle balsamic
  vinegar

8-ounce can grated fat-free or
  reduced-fat Parmesan

8-ounce can water chestnuts

10-ounce bottle soy sauce

12-ounce can fat-free
  breadcrumbs

12-ounce can fat-free panko
  (Japanese breadcrumbs)

16-ounce box regular couscous
16-ounce box raisins
16-ounce jar honey

16-ounce package angel-hair pasta
25-ounce jar applesauce, unsweetened

Produce

1 bunch basil
1 bunch celery
1 bunch chives
1 bunch cilantro
1 bunch scallions
1 head bok choy
1 head garlic
1 head romaine lettuce
1 orange
1 package broccoli florets
1 small piece fresh ginger
1 yellow bell pepper
2 medium yellow onions

2 medium russet potatoes
2 shallots
2 sweet potatoes
4 lemons
4 red bell peppers
6 Granny Smith apples
8 ounces snow peas
8 ounces sugar snap peas
8 portobello mushrooms
8-ounce package white button
mushrooms
10 large tomatoes

Week Three

Baking and Spices

1 bottle vanilla extract
1 box Old Bay Seasoning
1 can baking powder
1 can nonfat cooking spray
1 can salt
1 jar basil
1 jar black pepper
1 jar crushed red pepper flakes
1 jar curry powder
1 jar garlic salt
1 jar ground allspice

1 jar ground cinnamon
1 jar ground nutmeg
1 jar oregano
1 jar seasoning salt (preferably
Lawry's)
1 jar thyme
1-pound bag Splenda brown sugar
1-pound box cornstarch
5-pound bag all-purpose flour
5-pound bag whole-wheat flour
18-ounce can quick-cooking oats

Bread

1 package English muffins (6 count)
1 package wonton wrappers
  (50 count)

Dairy

1 carton fat-free cottage cheese
1 gallon fat-free milk
2 cartons fat-free ricotta
2 quarts Egg Beaters or 6 dozen
  eggs (for egg whites)
2 8-ounce packages fat-free
  shredded cheddar cheese
8-ounce package fat-free
  American cheese slices

8 ounces fat-free shredded
  mozzarella
8 ounces fat-free cream cheese

Frozen

1-pound bag blueberries
2 pounds individual frozen French bread dough loaves
3 10-ounce boxes chopped spinach

Meat and Shellfish

1 pound Canadian bacon
1 pound canned lump crabmeat
1 pound large shrimp
  (12–14 count)
2 pounds fresh littleneck clams

2½ pounds ground buffalo (3% fat)
4½ pounds boneless, skinless
  chicken breasts
12-ounce package lean turkey
  bacon

Other Staples and Condiments

1 box dry onion soup mix
1 jar fat-free mayonnaise
1 jar fat-free spaghetti sauce
1-pound bag chili lime chips,
  preferably Guiltless Gourmet

1 quart fat-free chicken broth
1 small jar all-fruit apricot jam
1 small bottle ketchup
1 small jar capers
4-ounce can pimentos

6-ounce can light tuna

6-ounce can tomato paste

8-ounce bottle balsamic vinegar

8-ounce box manicotti shells

8-ounce can fat-free or
  reduced-fat grated Parmesan

8-ounce can water chestnuts

10-ounce bottle soy sauce

12-ounce bottle cooking sherry

12-ounce can fat-free
  breadcrumbs

12-ounce can fat-free panko (Japanese breadcrumbs)

12 ounces angel-hair pasta

14-ounce can diced tomatoes

14-ounce can stewed tomatoes

15-ounce can tomato sauce

16-ounce box regular couscous

16-ounce jar honey

25-ounce jar applesauce, unsweetened

28-ounce can diced tomatoes

Produce

1 acorn squash

1 bunch basil

1 bunch cilantro

1 bunch dill

1 bunch flat-leaf parsley

1 bunch scallions

1 head garlic

1 head green-leaf lettuce

1 jalapeño pepper

1 mango

1 piece fresh ginger

1 plum tomato

2 medium red onions

2 medium zucchini

2 sweet potatoes

3 limes

5-ounce package baby spinach

6 medium yellow onions

7 large tomatoes

9 red bell peppers

12 ounces white button
  mushrooms

Week Four

Baking and Spices

1 bottle vanilla extract

1 box Old Bay Seasoning

1 can baking powder

1 can nonfat cooking spray

1 can salt

1 jar basil

1 jar black pepper

1 jar crushed red pepper flakes

1 jar cumin

1 jar curry powder

1 jar garlic salt
1 jar ground allspice
1 jar ground cinnamon
1 jar ground nutmeg
1 jar oregano
1 jar paprika
1 jar seasoning salt (preferably
Lawry's)

1 jar thyme
1-pound bag Splenda brown
sugar
1-pound box cornstarch
5-pound bag all-purpose flour
5-pound bag whole-wheat
flour
18-ounce can quick-cooking oats

Bread

1 loaf French or Italian bread
1 package 10-inch fat-free tortillas (10–12 count)
1 package 10-inch fat-free whole-wheat tortillas (10–12 count)
1 package pita bread (6 count)

Dairy

1 gallon fat-free milk
2 quarts Egg Beaters or 6 dozen eggs (for egg whites)
2 8-ounce packages fat-free cream cheese
2 8-ounce packages fat-free shredded cheddar cheese
8 ounces fat-free shredded mozzarella

Frozen

2 pounds French bread dough
12-ounce can orange juice concentrate

Meat, Fish, and Shellfish

1 pound canned lump crabmeat
3 pounds turkey breast
4 4-ounce center-cut pork loin
chops
6 pounds boneless, skinless
chicken breasts

6 ounces small shrimp
12-ounce package lean turkey
bacon
16 ounces tilapia fillets
24 ounces pork tenderloin

Other Staples and Condiments

1 bottle plum sauce (in Asian specialties section)

1 can fat-free evaporated milk

1 jar fat-free mayonnaise

1 jar hoisin sauce (in Asian specialties section)

1 jar roasted red peppers

1-pound bag chili lime chips, preferably Guiltless Gourmet

1 quart fat-free chicken broth

1 small can black olives

1 small jar all-fruit apricot jam

1 small jar capers

1 small jar pimentos

4-ounce can green chilies

6-ounce can tomato paste

8-ounce bottle balsamic vinegar

8-ounce can fat-free or reduced-fat Parmesan

8-ounce can water chestnuts

8-ounce jar green taco sauce

10-ounce bottle soy sauce

12-ounce bottle cooking sherry

12-ounce bottle rice wine vinegar

12-ounce bottle Worcestershire sauce

12-ounce can fat-free breadcrumbs

12-ounce can fat-free panko (Japanese breadcrumbs)

15-ounce can mandarin oranges in juice

16-ounce bottle fat-free ginger dressing, such as Newman's Own

16-ounce jar honey

16-ounce jar mild or medium salsa

16-ounce package angel-hair pasta

25-ounce jar applesauce, unsweetened

Produce

1 bunch basil

1 bunch celery

1 bunch chives

1 bunch cilantro

1 bunch flat-leaf parsley

1 bunch rosemary

1 bunch scallions

1 bunch thyme

1 carton white button mushrooms

1 head green leaf lettuce

1 head romaine lettuce

1 jalapeño pepper

1 small piece ginger

1 yellow bell pepper

2 Granny Smith apples

2 heads garlic

2 lemons

2 medium yellow onions

2 medium russet potatoes

2 shallots

3 limes

3 red bell peppers

4 Gala apples
8 ounces snow peas

8 portobello mushrooms
9 tomatoes

Week Five

BAKING AND SPICES

1 box Old Bay Seasoning
1 can baking powder
1 can nonfat cooking spray
1 can salt
1 jar basil
1 jar black pepper
1 jar cayenne pepper
1 jar chili powder
1 jar crushed red pepper flakes
1 jar cumin
1 jar curry powder
1 jar garlic salt

1 jar ground allspice
1 jar ground cinnamon
1 jar ground nutmeg
1 jar oregano
1 jar seasoning salt (preferably
   Lawry's)
1 jar thyme
1-pound bag Splenda brown sugar
1-pound box cornstarch
5-pound bag all-purpose flour
5-pound bag whole-wheat flour
18-ounce can quick-cooking oats

BREAD

1 loaf French or Italian bread
1 package English muffins (6 count)
1 package 10-inch fat-free whole-wheat tortillas (10–12 count)
1 package wonton wrappers (50 count)
2 packages 10-inch fat-free tortillas (10–12 count)

DAIRY

1 gallon fat-free milk
2 8-ounce packages fat-free cream
   cheese
2 15-ounce packages fat-free
   ricotta
2 quarts Egg Beaters or 6 dozen
   eggs (for egg whites)

12-ounce package fat-free
   American cheese slices
16 ounces fat-free shredded
   cheddar cheese

Frozen

1-pound bag blueberries
2 10-ounce boxes chopped spinach

Meat and Shellfish

1 pound Canadian bacon
1 pound large shrimp (12–14 count)
8 pounds boneless, skinless chicken breasts
8 8-ounce chicken breasts, bone in
12-ounce package lean turkey bacon

Other Staples and Condiments

1 jar fat-free mayonnaise
1-pound bag chili lime chips, preferably Guiltless Gourmet
1-pound package Splenda sugar
4-ounce can green chilies
8-ounce bottle picante sauce
8-ounce box manicotti shells
8-ounce can fat-free or reduced-fat Parmesan
8-ounce jar green taco sauce
12-ounce can fat-free breadcrumbs
12-ounce can fat-free panko (Japanese breadcrumbs)
15-ounce can mandarin oranges in juice
16-ounce bottle fat-free ginger dressing, such as Newman's Own
16-ounce jar honey
25-ounce jar applesauce, unsweetened
26-ounce jar fat-free spaghetti sauce

Produce

1 acorn squash
1 bunch basil
1 bunch dill
1 bunch Italian parsley
1 bunch scallions
1 bunch tarragon
1 bunch thyme
1 carton white button mushrooms
1 head romaine lettuce
1 mango
1 yellow bell pepper
2 bunches cilantro
2 heads garlic
2 heads green leaf lettuce

2 jalapeño peppers
2 limes
2 red bell peppers

4 large yellow onions
5-ounce bag baby spinach
8 large tomatoes

Week Six

Baking and Spices

1 bottle vanilla extract
1 box Old Bay Seasoning
1 can baking powder
1 can nonfat cooking spray
1 can salt
1 jar basil
1 jar black pepper
1 jar crushed red pepper flakes
1 jar curry powder
1 jar garlic salt
1 jar ground allspice
1 jar ground cinnamon

1 jar ground nutmeg
1 jar oregano
1 jar seasoning salt (preferably Lawry's)
1 jar thyme
1-pound bag Splenda brown sugar
1-pound box cornstarch
5-pound bag all-purpose flour
5-pound bag whole-wheat flour
16-ounce bottle light corn syrup
18-ounce can quick-cooking oats

Bread

1 loaf French or Italian bread
1 package English muffins (6 count)
1 package 10-inch fat-free tortillas (10–12 count)
1 package 10-inch fat-free whole-wheat tortillas (10–12 count)
1 package pita bread (6 count)

Dairy

1 gallon fat-free milk
2 quarts Egg Beaters or 6 dozen eggs (for egg whites)
2 8-ounce packages fat-free shredded cheddar cheese

8 ounces fat-free cream cheese
8 ounces fat-free shredded mozzarella
15 ounces fat-free ricotta

FROZEN

1-pound bag blueberries
1 pound frozen French bread dough
12-ounce can orange juice concentrate

MEAT AND SHELLFISH

1 pound canned lump
   crabmeat
1 pound bay or sea scallops
1 pound Canadian bacon
2 pounds littleneck clams

4 4-ounce center-cut pork loin
   chops
5½ pounds boneless, skinless
   chicken breasts
12 ounces pork tenderloin

OTHER STAPLES AND CONDIMENTS

1 bottle marsala cooking wine
1 can fat-free evaporated milk
1 jar fat-free mayonnaise
1 jar roasted red peppers
1 quart fat-free chicken broth
1 small jar all-fruit apricot jam
1 small jar capers
4-ounce can green chilies
6-ounce can tomato paste
8-ounce bottle balsamic vinegar
8-ounce can fat-free or reduced-
   fat Parmesan
8-ounce can water chestnuts
10-ounce bottle soy sauce
12-ounce bottle cooking sherry
12-ounce bottle rice wine vinegar
12-ounce bottle Worcestershire
   sauce

12-ounce can fat-free
   breadcrumbs
12-ounce can fat-free panko (Japanese breadcrumbs)
12 ounces angel-hair pasta
14-ounce can diced tomatoes
15-ounce can mandarin oranges in
   juice
16-ounce bottle fat-free ginger
   dressing, such as Paul
   Newman's
16-ounce box raisins
16-ounce box regular
   couscous
16-ounce jar honey
16-ounce jar mild or medium salsa
28-ounce can diced tomatoes

PRODUCE

1 bunch basil
1 bunch celery
1 bunch chives
1 bunch cilantro
1 bunch dill
1 bunch parsley
1 bunch scallions
1 head romaine lettuce
1 orange
1 plum tomato
1 yellow bell pepper
1 zucchini
2 Granny Smith apples

2 heads garlic
2 medium red onions
2 medium yellow onions
2 russet potatoes
2 sweet potatoes
4 Gala apples
4 lemons
5-ounce bag baby spinach
5 large tomatoes
8 ounces white button mushrooms
8 portobello mushrooms
12 red bell peppers

Appetizers, Dips, Sauces, Side Dishes, Soups, and Salads

Please note that specific quantities are omitted in the following section for spices, condiments, and various staples that you may already have purchased as part of the weekly shopping lists. If you have any questions, please refer to the original recipe.

ALL CHOKED UP ARTICHOKE DIP

1 bunch flat-leaf parsley
1 bunch scallions
2 ounces fat-free ricotta
2 ounces fat-free sour cream

19-ounce can artichoke hearts
Fat-free mayonnaise
Garlic
Grated fat-free Parmesan

ALL CURRIED UP DIP/SPREAD

1 large sweet onion
2 15-ounce containers fat-free ricotta
Curry powder

All Steamed Up Artichokes

1 lemon
4 large artichokes

Asparagus with Dip

2 pounds fresh asparagus
Curry powder
Fat-free mayonnaise
Garlic

Baked Light French Fries

6 large russet potatoes
Garlic salt
Nonfat cooking spray
Seasoning salt (preferably Lawry's)

Baked Potato Latkes

2 medium yellow onions
2 pounds russet potatoes
All-purpose flour
Egg Beaters or 3 eggs (for egg
   whites)

Nonfat cooking spray
Seasoning salt
   (preferably Lawry's)

Barbecue Sauce

8 ounces ketchup
Chili powder
Cumin

Soy sauce
Splenda brown sugar
Worcestershire sauce

Blue-Stuffed Tomatoes

1 pound broccoli florets
4 large tomatoes

Fat-free blue cheese dressing
Grated fat-free Parmesan
Instant stuffing mix, herb flavor

BRUSCHETTA, ANYONE?

1 bunch basil
1 bunch oregano
1 French baguette
1 large onion (any variety)

3 large tomatoes
Garlic
Grated fat-free Parmesan
Nonfat cooking spray

CANDIED CARROTS

1 lemon
1 pound large carrots
1 small piece fresh ginger
Raisins
Splenda brown sugar

CHEESY BROCCOLI BAKE

1 medium yellow onion
2 pounds broccoli florets
8 ounces fat-free milk
12 ounces shredded fat-free
   cheddar cheese

Nonfat cooking spray
Egg Beaters

CREAMY MUSHROOM SOUP

4 ounces fat-free milk
20 ounces nonfat beef or chicken
   stock
1 medium yellow onion
1 medium russet potato

14 ounces white button mush-
   rooms
Cooking sherry
Garlic
Nonfat cooking spray

CRISPY PANKO SHRIMP APPETIZERS

1 pound large shrimp (12 to 14 count)
Cornstarch
Egg Beaters or 2 eggs (for egg whites)
Fat-free panko (Japanese breadcrumbs)
Nonfat cooking spray
Seasoning salt (preferably Lawry's)
White pepper

CURRIED CAULIFLOWER BAKE

2 pounds cauliflower
3 ounces fat-free plain yogurt
Cumin
Curry powder
Fat-free breadcrumbs
Grated fat-free Parmesan
Nonfat cooking spray
Turmeric

EASIEST RICE PILAF EVER

1 small yellow onion
8 ounces white rice
14 ounces fat-free chicken stock
Bay leaf
Nonfat cooking spray

FALL FRUIT WITH VANILLA MAPLE DIP

1 large apple
1 large pear
1 lemon
1 pound green grapes
1 small bottle sugar-free maple syrup
16 ounces fat-free vanilla yogurt

FINE HERB SAUCE

1 bunch basil
1 bunch oregano
1 bunch thyme
Cooking sherry

Green Bean Casserole

1 medium yellow onion

4 ounces shredded fat-free
cheddar cheese

9-ounce package frozen
French-style green beans

10-ounce can fat-free cream of
mushroom soup

28-ounce can Durkee's
French-fried Onions

Nonfat cooking spray

Guiltless Mac and Cheese

4 ounces shredded fat-free
cheddar cheese

8 ounces fat-free milk

8 ounces elbow macaroni

12 ounces fat-free, small-curd
cottage cheese

All-purpose flour

Dried mustard

Fat-free breadcrumbs

Grated fat-free Parmesan or
Romano

Nonfat cooking spray

Herb-Roasted Vegetables

1 bunch basil

1 bunch flat-leaf parsley

1 bunch thyme

1 medium red onion

1 red bell pepper

2 bunches broccoli

4 ounces fat-free chicken stock

8 ounces large carrots

16 ounces white button
mushrooms

Balsamic or apple cider
vinegar

Garlic

Grated fat-free Parmesan

Italian Vegetable Salad

1 red bell pepper

1 medium red onion

1 yellow bell pepper

2 English cucumbers

4 plum tomatoes

2 ounces fat-free feta

Black pepper

Fat-free Italian dressing

Joe's Wild, Wild Mushroom Risotto

1 bunch thyme
1 small yellow onion
4 ounces Arborio rice
4 ounces cremini mushrooms
4 ounces shiitake mushrooms

4 ounces white button
    mushrooms
12 ounces fat-free chicken stock
Garlic
Nonfat cooking spray

Leek and Gold Potato Soup

1 large yellow onion
1 quart fat-free chicken broth
2 large leeks
8 Yukon gold potatoes

Mexican Spring Rolls

1 bunch cilantro
1 bunch scallions
4-ounce can chopped green
    chilies
1 jicama
1 pound chicken tenders

2 limes
12 round 8-inch rice papers
    (available in Asian specialties
    section)
16 ounces orange juice
Cumin

No Crying Onion Quesadillas

1 bunch cilantro
1 jalapeño pepper
1 large Vidalia or sweet onion
4 7-inch fat-free flour tortillas

6 ounces shredded fat-free
    mozzarella or Monterey jack
Nonfat cooking spray

No-Fry Sweet Potato French Fries

2 large sweet potatoes
Cayenne pepper
Chili powder
Grated fat-free Parmesan

ROASTED CANDIED ACORN SQUASH

1 small piece fresh ginger
2 acorn squashes
Ground allspice
Nonfat cooking spray
Splenda brown sugar

ROASTED CARAMELIZED ONIONS

4 large Vidalia or sweet onions
Balsamic vinegar
Dried thyme
Notfat cooking spray
Splenda brown sugar

ROASTED GARLIC HUMMUS

1 bunch flat-leaf parsley
1 lemon
1 medium red onion
2 8-ounce cans garbanzo beans

2 heads garlic
Cayenne pepper
Nonfat cooking spray

SOUTH OF THE BORDER DIP

1 lime
1 red bell pepper
1 small red onion
1 small tomato

8 ounces fat-free refried beans
Chili powder
Cumin
Garlic

SOUTHWESTERN CHEESE DIP

1 or 2 jalapeño peppers
1 red bell pepper
1 yellow bell pepper
8 ounces fat-free cream cheese

Chili powder
Cumin
Garlic salt

SPINACH DIP

1 bunch flat-leaf parsley
4 ounces fat-free plain yogurt
5 ounces fresh spinach

6 ounces fat-free cream cheese
Garlic
Grated fat-free Parmesan

SPINACH, RASPBERRY AND MANDARIN ORANGE SALAD

1 medium red onion
1 pint raspberries
1 pound baby spinach
4 ounces white button mushrooms

15-ounce can mandarin orange
    slices in juice
Fat-free raspberry salad
    dressing

SWEET POTATO KUGEL

1 medium carrot
1 medium russet potato
1 pound sweet potatoes
12-ounce can orange juice
    concentrate

Egg Beaters
Fat-free breadcrumbs
Golden raisins
Ground allspice
Nonfat cooking spray

SWEET AND SOUR COLESLAW

1 bunch scallions
1 head green cabbage
1 head red cabbage
1 small piece fresh ginger
1 yellow bell pepper
6 ounces snow peas

8 ounces water chestnuts
Fat-free mayonnaise
Garlic
Rice wine vinegar
Soy sauce
Splenda brown sugar

SWEET AND SPICY TURKEY PINWHEELS

1 bunch scallions
1 bunch spinach
3 ounces canned mandarin
    oranges in juice
4 10-inch fat-free flour tortillas

4 ounces fat-free cream cheese
6 ounces low-fat or fat-free
    smoked turkey, thinly sliced
Cumin

Sweet and Tart Carrots and Apples

1 pound baby carrots
4 large Granny Smith apples
3 ounces dried tart cherries

Ground cinnamon
Nonfat cooking spray
Splenda brown sugar

Up in Smoke Turkey Spread

1 bunch cilantro
8 ounces fat-free cream cheese
8 ounces smoked turkey
Cayenne pepper

Wild Mushroom Crostini

1 French baguette
1 bunch thyme
2 shallots
4 ounces shiitake mushrooms

4 ounces fat-free cream cheese
8 ounces cremini mushrooms
Nonfat cooking spray

Zucchini Fingers

4 small zucchini
Egg Beaters or 4 eggs (for egg
  whites)
Grated fat-free Parmesan

Nonfat cooking spray
Panko (Japanese breadcrumbs)
Seasoning salt
  (preferably Lawry's)

Snacks

Air-popped popcorn
Apple Cinnamon Quaker Rice
  Cakes
Beef jerky
Caramel Corn Quaker Rice Cakes
Fat-free muffins

Fat-free pretzels
Fig Newman's
Fruit—remember to buy a variety
  for healthy snacking
No Pudge Brownies
Raisin

Appendix 2

The Sierras Solution
Decision Balance Sheet

Name: Date:
_____

What I'm trying to decide:
_____

Good Things About Doing This

1. _____
2. _____
3. _____
4. _____
5. _____
6. _____
7. _____
8. _____

Challenging Things About Doing This

1. _____
2. _____
3. _____
4. _____
5. _____
6. _____
7. _____
8. _____

Appendix 3

The Sierras Solution
Goal Sheet

Name: Date:

_____

From _____ to _____, I will do the following:

_____

1. _____
2. _____
3. _____
   _____

                                    _____
                                              Signature

Appendix 4

The Sierras Solution
Activity Plan

Name: _____ From _____ to _____
(Dates)

1. STEPS PER DAY—GOALS:
   Minimum Goal: 10,000

   My Goal: _____

   Plans for Achieving My Goal:

   _____

   _____

2. WORKOUT ACTIVITIES—GOALS:

   My Goal: _____

   Plans for Achieving My Goal:

   _____

   _____

3. MINIMIZING SEDENTARY BEHAVIORS—GOALS:

My Goal: _____

Plans for Achieving My Goal:

_____

_____

4. SOURCES OF ENCOURAGEMENT:

_____

_____

5. METHODS OF PROBLEM SOLVING:

_____

_____

Appendix 5

The Sierras Solution
Self-Monitoring Journal (SMJ)

Day:	Mon. Tues. Wed. Thurs. Fri. Sat. Sun.

Date: _____

STEPS: _____ EXERCISE _____

Time	Food	Calories	Fat Grams
	TOTALS:		

MOVEMENT AND ACTIVITIES

Rating (0–100; 100 =
goals reached + maximum effort):

THINK AND INK

LINK:

Appendix 5:
The Sierras
Solution
Self-Monitoring
Journal (SMJ)

328

Appendix 6

Calculating Body Mass Index

In order to calculate body mass index (BMI) by hand and determine the BMI percentile without the use of the Internet, do the following calculation:

1. Find your or your weight controller's BMI by calculating

Your weight in pounds ÷ (Your height in inches)^2 × 703 = Your BMI.

For example, a sixteen-year-old boy who is 68 inches tall and weighs 190 pounds would work out to: $190 ÷ 68^2 = 190 ÷ 4624 = .041 × 703 = 28.9$ BMI.

2. For your weight controller, use the following BMI charts to determine the BMI percentile. For this example, the BMI percentile is >95 percent.

3. Select a reasonable weight goal for yourself for the next year and recalculate your target BMI accordingly. For your weight controller, guess how much your child will grow in the next year and recalculate the BMI accordingly. Then look up his or her new BMI percentile.

In this example, a weight loss of twenty pounds, combined with an assumed 1-inch increase in height over the course of a year (making the boy seventeen years old), would yield:

$170 \div 69^2 = 170 \div 4761 = .036 \times 703 = 25.3$ BMI.

Since he would have aged one year while losing the weight, he would look at the data for seventeen-year-olds. His BMI percentile would be 87.

4. Check the list below to see if your target BMI is within normal range.

BMI	WEIGHT STATUS
Below 18.5	Underweight
18.5–24.9	Normal
25.0–29.9	Overweight
30.0+	Obese

If not, revise your goal accordingly, keeping in mind that your weight loss will average one-half to one pound a week.

For your weight controller, continue to revise the weight goal until you get below the 85th percentile. In the sample case, just adding another five pounds to the goal would do it. You could keep that twenty-five-pound goal or use a less aggressive goal, like fifteen pounds. In either case, achieving such goals in a year would make a big difference in health and appearance.

2 to 20 years: Girls
Body mass index-for-age percentiles

NAME _____

RECORD # _____

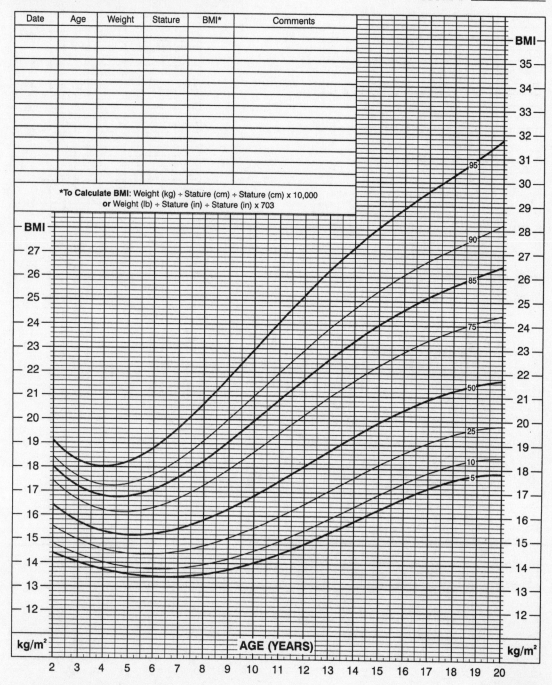

Date	Age	Weight	Stature	BMI*	Comments

*To Calculate BMI: Weight (kg) ÷ Stature (cm) ÷ Stature (cm) x 10,000
or Weight (lb) ÷ Stature (in) ÷ Stature (in) x 703

BMI

35
34
33
32
31
30
29
28
27
26
25
24
23
22
21
20
19
18
17
16
15
14
13
12

95
90
85
75
50
25
10
5

BMI

27
26
25
24
23
22
21
20
19
18
17
16
15
14
13
12

kg/m²

AGE (YEARS)

2 3 4 5 6 7 8 9 10 11 12 13 14 15 16 17 18 19 20

kg/m²

Published May 30, 2000 (modified 10/16/00).
SOURCE: Developed by the National Center for Health Statistics in collaboration with
the National Center for Chronic Disease Prevention and Health Promotion (2000).
http://www.cdc.gov/growthcharts

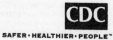

CDC
SAFER · HEALTHIER · PEOPLE™

2 to 20 years: Boys
Body mass index-for-age percentiles

NAME _____

RECORD # _____

Date	Age	Weight	Stature	BMI*	Comments

*To Calculate BMI: Weight (kg) ÷ Stature (cm) ÷ Stature (cm) x 10,000
or Weight (lb) ÷ Stature (in) ÷ Stature (in) x 703

BMI

35
34
33
32
31
30
95
29
28
90
27
85
26
25
75
24
23
50
22
21
25
20
10
19
5
18
17
16
15
14
13
12

BMI

27
26
25
24
23
22
21
20
19
18
17
16
15
14
13
12

kg/m²   AGE (YEARS)   kg/m²

2 3 4 5 6 7 8 9 10 11 12 13 14 15 16 17 18 19 20

Published May 30, 2000 (modified 10/16/00).
SOURCE: Developed by the National Center for Health Statistics in collaboration with
the National Center for Chronic Disease Prevention and Health Promotion (2000).
http://www.cdc.gov/growthcharts

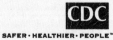

SAFER · HEALTHIER · PEOPLE™

References

Chapter One: The Sierras Solution

Dietz, W. H., and T. N. Robinson. 2005. Overweight children and adolescents. *New England Journal of Medicine* 352:2100–2109.

Braet, C. 2006. Patient characteristics as predictors of weight loss after an obesity treatment for children. *Obesity* 14:148–155.

Hedley, A. A., et al. 2004. Prevalence of overweight and obesity among U.S. children, adolescents, and adults, 1999–2002. *Journal of the American Medical Association* 291:2847–2850.

Nader, P. R., et al. 2006. Identifying risk for obesity in early childhood. *Pediatrics* 118:e594–e601.

Ogden, C. L., et al. 2002. Prevalence and trends in overweight among U.S. children and adolescents, 1999–2000. *Journal of the American Medical Association* 288:1728–1732.

Powell, L. H. and J. E. Calvin. 2007. Effective obesity treatments. *American Psychologist* 62:234–246.

Schwimmer, J. B., T. M. Burwinkle, and J. W. Varni. 2003. Health-related quality of life of severely obese children and adolescents. *Journal of the American Medical Association* 289:1813–1819.

Wadden, T. A., and A. J. Stunkard, eds. 2002. *Handbook of Obesity Treatment*. New York: Guilford Press.

Wang, Y., and T. Lobstein. 2006. Worldwide trends in childhood and adolescent obesity. *International Journal of Pediatric Obesity* 1:11–25.

Chapter Two: Why Kids Gain Weight

Barnard, N. D., A. Akhtar, and A. Nicholson. 1995. Factors that facilitate compliance to lower fat intake. *Archives of Family Medicine* 4:153–158.

Bessesen, D. H., C. L. Rupp, and R. H. Eckel. 1995. Dietary fat is shunted away from oxidation, toward storage in obese Zucker rats. *Obesity Research* 3:179–189.

Blass, E. 1989. Opioids, sweets, and a mechanism for positive affect: Broad motivational implications. In J. Dobbing, ed. *Sweetness.* New York: Springer-Verlag.

Blundell, J. E., V. J. Burley, J. R. Cotton, and C. L. Lawton. 1993. Dietary fat in the control of energy intake: Evaluating the effects of fat on meal size and postmeal satiety. *American Journal of Clinical Nutrition* 57:772S–778S.

Boozer, C. N., A. Brasseur, and R. L. Atkinson. 1993. Dietary fat affects weight loss and adiposity during energy restriction in rats. *American Journal of Clinical Nutrition* 58:846–852.

Brownell, K. D., and K. B. Horgen. 2004. *Food fight.* Chicago: Contemporary Books.

Critser, G. 2004. *Fat land.* Boston: Mariner.

Dobbing, J., ed. 1987. *Sweetness.* New York: Springer-Verlag.

Epstein, L. H., A. Valoski, R. R., Wing, and J. McCurley. 1994. Ten-year outcomes of behavioral family-based treatment for childhood obesity. *Health Psychology* 13:373–383.

Geiselman, P. J., and D. Novin. 1982. The role of carbohydrates in appetite, hunger and obesity. *Appetite* 3:203–223.

Hartigan, K. J., D. Baker-Strauch, and G. W. Morris. 1982. Perceptions of the causes of obesity and responsiveness to treatment. *Journal of Counseling Psychology* 29:478–485.

Hill, J. O., H. Drougas, and J. C. Peters. 1993. Obesity treatment: Can diet composition play a role? *Annals of Internal Medicine* 119:694–697.

Jeffery, R. W., W. L. Hellerstedt, S. A. French, and J. E. Baxter. 1995. A randomized trial of counseling for fat restriction versus calorie restriction in the treatment of obesity. *International Journal of Obesity* 19:132–137.

Jeffery, R. W., R. R. Wing, and R. R. Mayer. 1998. Are smaller weight losses or more achievable weight loss goals better in the long term for obese patients? *Journal of Consulting and Clinical Psychology* 66:641–645.

Kirschenbaum, D. S., et al. 1992. Stages of change in successful weight control: A clinically derived model. *Behavior Therapy* 23:623–635.

Kramer, F. M., R. W. Jeffery, J. L. Forster, and M. K. Snell. 1989. Long-term follow-up of behavioral treatment for obesity: Patterns of weight regain among men and women. *International Journal of Obesity* 13:123–136.

Liebman, B. 2004. Fat: More than just a lump of lard. *Nutrition Action Health Letter* 31:1–6.

Ravussin, E., and B. A. Swinburn. 1993. Energy metabolism. In A. J. Stunkard and T. A. Wadden, eds. *Obesity: Theory & therapy.* 2nd ed. New York: Raven Press.

Sims, E.Z.H., E. Danforth, et al. 1973. Endocrine and metabolic effects of experimental obesity in man. *Recent Progress in Hormone Research* 29:457–487.

Stunkard, A. J. 1958. The management of obesity. *New York State Journal of Medicine* 58:79–87.

Wadden, T. A., 1993. Treatment of obesity by moderate and severe caloric restriction: Results of clinical research trials. *Annals of Internal Medicine* 119:688–693.

Wadden, T. A., et al. 1997. Lifestyle modification in the pharmacologic treatment of obesity: A pilot investigation of a potential primary care approach. *Obesity Research* 5:218–226.

Weight-loss news that's easy to stomach. 1996. *Tufts University Diet & Nutrition Letter* 14.

Chapter 3: Nurture the Desire to Change

Hubbel, M. A., B. L. Duncan, and S. D. Miller, eds. 1999. *The heart and soul of change: What works in therapy*. Washington, DC: American Psychological Association.

Janis, I. L., and L. Mann. 1977. *Decision making: A psychological analysis of conflict, choice, and commitment*. New York: The Free Press.

Kirsch, I. 1990. *Changing expectations: A key to effective psychotherapy*. Pacific Grove, CA: Brooks/Cole.

Kirschenbaum, D. S., M. L. Fitzgibbon, S. Martino, J. H. Conviser, E. H. Rosendahl, and L. Laatsch. 1992. Stages of change in successful weight control: A clinically derived model. *Behavior Therapy* 23:623–635.

Meichenbaum, D., and D. C. Turk. 1987. *Facilitating treatment adherence: A practitioner's guidebook*. New York: Plenum.

Nelson, L. R., and M. L. Furst. 1972. An objective study of the effects of expectation on competitive performance. *Journal of Psychology* 81:69–72.

Shapiro, A. K. 1978. Placebo effects in medicine, psychotherapy, and psychoanalysis. In A. P. Bergin and S. L. Garfield, eds. *Handbook of psychotherapy and behavior change: An empirical analysis*. New York: John Wiley.

Vincent, P. 1971. Factors influencing patient noncompliance: A theoretical approach. *Nursing Research* 20:509–516.

Wang, S. S., S. Houshyar, and M. J. Prinstein. 2006. Adolescent girls' and boys' weight-related health behaviors and cognitions: Associations with reputation- and preference-based peer status. *Health Psychology* 25:658–663.

Wadden, T. A., L. G. Womble, A. J. Stunkard, and D. A. Anderson. 2002. Psychosocial consequences of obesity and weight loss. In T. A. Wadden and A. J. Stunkard, eds. *Handbook of Obesity Treatment*. New York: Guilford Press.

Chapter 4: Navigate the Six Stages of Change

Hubbel, M. A., B. L. Duncan, and S. D. Miller, eds. 1999. *The heart and soul of change: What works in therapy*. Washington, DC: American Psychological Association.

Ikemi, Y., and S. Nakagawa. 1962. A psychosomatic study of contagious dermatitis. *Kyosu Journal of Medical Science* 13:335–350.

Janis, I. L., and L. Mann, 1977. *Decision making: A psychological analysis of conflict, choice, and commitment*. New York: The Free Press.

Kirsch, I. 1990. *Changing expectations: A key to effective psychotherapy*. Pacific Grove, CA: Brooks/Cole.

Kirschenbaum, D. S., M. L. Fitzgibbon, S. Martino, J. H. Conviser, E. H. Rosendahl, and L. Laatsch. 1992. Stages of change in successful weight control: A clinically derived model. *Behavior Therapy* 23:623–635.

Meichenbaum, D., and D. C. Turk. 1987. *Facilitating treatment adherence: A practitioner's guidebook*. New York: Plenum.

Nelson, L. R., and M. L. Furst. 1972. An objective study of the effects of expectation on competitive performance. *Journal of Psychology* 81:69–72.

Shapiro, A. K. 1978. Placebo effects in medicine, psychotherapy, and psychoanalysis. In A. P. Bergin and S. L. Garfield, eds. *Handbook of psychotherapy and behavior change: An empirical analysis*. New York: John Wiley.

Vincent, P. 1971. Factors influencing patient noncompliance: A theoretical approach. *Nursing Research* 20:509–516.

Chapter 5: Help Your Child Manage Stress

Alberti, R. E., and M. L. Emmons. 1990. *Your perfect right: A guide to assertive living*. 6th ed. San Luis Obispo, CA: Impact Publishers.

Barlow, D. H., and R. M. Rapee. 1991. *Mastering stress. A lifestyle approach*. Dallas: American Health Publishing.

Bourne, E. J. 1990. *The anxiety and phobia workbook*. Oakland, CA: New Harbinger Publications.

Burns, D. E. 1989. *The feeling good handbook: Using the new mood therapy in everyday life*. New York: William Morrow.

Cautela, J. R., and J. Groden. 1991. *Relaxation: A comprehensive manual for adults, children, and children with special needs*. Champaign, IL: Research Press.

Davis, M., E. R. Eshelman, and M. McKay. 1995. *The relaxation and stress reduction workbook*. 4th ed. Oakland, CA: New Harbinger Publications.

Ellis, A., and R. A. Harper. 1975. *A new guide to rational living*. Hollywood, CA: Wilshire Book Co.

Grasha, A. F., and D. S. Kirschenbaum. 1986. *Adjustment and competence: Concepts and applications*. Minneapolis: West Publishing.

Harp, D., with N. Feldman. 1990. *The new three minute mediator*. Oakland, CA: New Harbinger Publications.

Holmes, T. H., and R. H. Rahe. 1967. The social readjustment rating scale. *Journal of Psychosomatic Research* 11:216.

Jacobson, E. 1929. *Progressive relaxation*. Chicago: University of Chicago Press.

Kirschenbaum, D. S., and D. A. Wittrock. 1990. Still searching for effective criticism inoculation procedures. *Journal of Applied Sport Psychology* 2:175–185.

Marks, I. M. 1978. *Living with fear: Understanding and coping with anxiety*. New York: McGraw-Hill.

Meichenbaum, D. 1985. *Stress inoculation training*. New York: Pergamon.

Stevens, J. O. 1971. *Awareness: Exploring, experimenting, experiencing*. Moab, UT: Real People Press.

Thayer, R. E. 1987. Energy, tiredness, and tension effects of a sugar snack versus moderate exercise. *Journal of Personality and Social Psychology* 52:119–125.

Tubesing, N. L., and D. H. Tubesing. 1990. *Structured exercises in stress management*. Vols. 1–4. Duluth, MN: Whole Person Press.

Zilberg, N. J., D. S. Weiss, and M. J. Horowitz. 1982. Impact of event scale: A cross-validation study. *Journal of Consulting and Clinical Psychology* 50:407–414.

Chapter 6: The Three Simple Changes

Brehm, J. W. 1966. *A theory of psychological reactance*. New York: Academic Press.

Goldman, G. 1978. Contract teaching of academic skills. *Journal of Consulting and Clinical Psychology* 25:320–324.

Locke, E. A., and G. P. Latham. 1990. *A theory of goal setting and task performance*. Englewood Cliffs, NJ: Prentice Hall.

Smith, H. W. 1994. *The ten natural laws of time and life management*. New York: Warner.

Weinberg, R. S., and D. Gould. 2006. *Foundations of sport and exercise psychology*. 4th ed. Champaign, IL: Human Kinetics.

Chapter 7: Simple Change #1—Eat Fewer than 20 Fat Grams Per Day

Agatston, A. 2003. *The South Beach diet: The delicious, doctor-designed, foolproof plan for fast and healthy weight loss*. Emmaus, PA: Rodale Press.

Atkins, R. C. 1998. *Dr. Atkins' new diet revolution*. New York: Avon Books.

Barnard, N. D., A. Akhtar, and A. Nicholson. 1995. Factors that facilitate compliance to lower fat intake. *Archives of Family Medicine* 4:153–158.

Bessesen, D. H., C. L. Rupp, and R. H. Eckel. 1995. Dietary fat is shunted away from oxidation, toward storage in obese Zucker rats. *Obesity Research* 3:179–189.

Boozer, C. N., A. Brasseur, and Atkinson, R. L. 1993. Dietary fat affects weight loss and adiposity during energy restriction in rats. *American Journal of Clinical Nutrition* 58:846–852.

Fleming, R. M. 2002. The effect of high-, moderate-, and low-fat diets on weight loss and cardiovascular disease risk factors. *Preventive Cardiology* 5:110–118.

Harris, J. K., S. A. French, R. W. Jeffery, P. McGovern, and R. R. Wing. 1994. Dietary and physical activity correlates of long-term weight loss. *Obesity Research* 2:307–313.

Kirschenbaum, D. S. 2005. Very low-fat diets are much better than low-carbohydrate diets: A position paper based on science. *Patient Care* 39:47–55.

Mann, T., A. J. Tomiyana, et al. 2007. Medicare's search for effective obesity treatments: Diets are not the answer. *American Psychologist* 62:220–233.

Rozin, P., M. Ashmore, and M. Markwith. 1996. Lay conceptions of nutrition: Dose insensitivity, categorical thinking, contagion, and the monotonic mind. *Health Psychology* 15:438–447.

Sears, B., and B. Lawren. 1995. *The zone: A dietary road map to lose weight permanently, reset your genetic code, prevent disease, achieve maximum physical performance.* New York: HarperCollins.

Stice, E. 1998. Prospective relation of dieting behaviors to weight change in a community sample of adolescents. *Behavior Therapy* 29:277–297.

Van Horn, L., and R. E. Kavey. 1997. Diet and cardiovascular disease prevention: What works? *Annals of Behavioral Medicine* 19:197–212.

Wadden, T. A., and S. Osei. 2002. The treatment of obesity: An overview. In T. A. Wadden and A. J. Stunkard, eds. *Handbook of obesity treatment.* New York: Guilford Press.

Weigle, D. S., D. E. Cummings, et al. 2003. Roles of leptin and ghrelin in the loss of body weight caused by a low fat, high carbohydrate diet. *Journal of Clinical and Endocrinological Metabolism* 88:1577–1586.

Chapter 8: Simple Change #2: Take at Least Ten Thousand Steps Every Day

Baechle, T. R., and B. R. Groves. 1992. *Weight training: Steps to success.* Champaign, IL: Leisure Press.

Blair, S. N. 1991. *Living with exercise.* Dallas: American Health Publishing.

———.1991. Weight loss through physical activity. *Weight Control Digest* 1:17, 20–24.

Carpenter, R. A. 2004. Getting in step with counters. *Weight Management Newsletter of the American Dietetic Association* 1:1–2.

Curless, M. R. 1992. Only the fit stay young. *Self*, September:180–181.

Dishman, R. K., ed. 1988. *Exercise adherence: Its impact on public health.* Champaign, IL: Human Kinetics Publishers.

Donahoe, C. P., Jr., D. H. Lin, D. S. Kirschenbaum, and R. E. Keesey. 1984. Metabolic consequences of dieting and exercise in the treatment of obesity. *Journal of Consulting and Clinical Psychology* 52:827–836.

Galvin, J. 1991. *The exercise habit: Your personal road map to developing a lifelong exercise commitment.* Champaign, IL: Human Kinetics Publishers.

Heil, J. 1993. *Psychology of sport injury.* Champaign, IL: Human Kinetics Publishers.

Kendzierski, D., and W. Johnson. 1993. Excuses, excuses, excuses: A cognitive behavioral approach to exercise implementation. *Journal of Sport and Exercise Psychology* 15:207–219.

Kirschenbaum, D. S. 1998. *Mind matters: Seven steps to smarter sport performance.* Carmel, IN: Cooper Publishing Group.

Kusinitz, I., M. Fin, and Editors of Consumer Reports Books. 1983. *Physical fitness for practically everybody: The Consumer's Union report on exercise*. Mount Vernon, NY: Consumer's Union.

Latella, F. S., W. Conkling, and Editors of Consumer Reports Books. 1989. *Get in shape, stay in shape*. Mount Vernon, NY: Consumer Reports Books.

Rippe, J. M., and P. Amend. 1992. *The exercise exchange program*. New York: Simon & Schuster.

Vickery, S., and M. Moffat. 1999. *The American Physical Therapy Association book of body repair and maintenance*. New York: Owl Books.

Chapter 9: Simple Change #3: Self-Monitor Every Day

Baker, R. C., and D. S. Kirschenbaum. 1993. Self-monitoring may be necessary for successful weight control. *Behavior Therapy* 24:377–394.

———. 1998. Weight control during the holidays: Highly consistent self-monitoring as a potentially useful coping mechanism. *Health Psychology*, 17:367–370.

Baumeister, R. F., T. F. Heatherton, and D. M. Tice. 1994. *Losing control: How and why people fail at self-regulation*. San Diego: Academic Press.

Boutelle, K. N., and D. S. Kirschenbaum. 1998. Further support for consistent self-monitoring as a vital component of successful weight control. *Obesity Research* 6:219–224.

Boutelle, K. N., D. S. Kirschenbaum, R. C. Baker, and M. E. Mitchell. 1999. How can obese weight controllers minimize weight gain during the high-risk holiday season? By self-monitoring very consistently. *Health Psychology* 18:364–368.

Carver, C. S., and M. F. Scheier. 1990. Origins and functions of positive and negative affect: A control-process view. *Psychological Review* 97:19–35.

Kanfer, F. H., and P. Karoly. 1972. Self-control: A behavioristic excursion into the lion's den. *Behavior Therapy* 3:398–416.

Kirschenbaum, D. S. 1987. Self-regulatory failure: A review with clinical implications. *Clinical Psychology Review* 7:77–104.

Kirschenbaum, D. S., J. N. Germann, and B. H. Rich. 2005. Treatment of morbid obesity in low-income minority adolescents: Participant and parental self-monitoring as determinants of initial success. *Obesity Research* 13:1527–1529.

Perri, M. G., A. M. Nezu, and B. J. Viegener. 1992. *Improving the long-term management of obesity: Theory, research, and clinical guidelines*. New York: John Wiley.

Schlundt, D. G., T. Sbrocco, and C. Bell. 1989. Identification of high-risk situations in a behavioral weight-loss program: Application of the relapse prevention model. *International Journal of Obesity* 13:223–234.

Sperduto, W. A., H. S. Thompson, and R. M. O'Brien. 1986. The effect of target behavior monitoring on weight loss and completion rate in a behavior modification program for weight reduction. *Addictive Behaviors* 11:337–340.

Weinberg, R. S. 1988. *The mental advantage: Developing your psychological skills in tennis*. Champaign, IL: Leisure Press.

Chapter 10: Encourage a Healthy Obsession

Baker, R. C., and D. S. Kirschenbaum. 1998. Weight control during the holidays: Highly consistent self-monitoring as a potentially useful coping mechanism. *Health Psychology* 17:367–370.

Barnard, N. D., A. Akhtar, and A. Nicholson. 1995. Factors that facilitate compliance to lower fat intake. *Archives of Family Medicine* 4:153–158.

Braet, C., and M. Van Winckel. 2000. Long-term follow-up of a cognitive behavioral treatment program for obese children. *Behavior Therapy* 31:55–74.

Baumeister, R. F., T. F. Heatherton, and D. M. Tice. 1994. *Losing control: How and why people fail at self-regulation*. San Diego: Academic Press.

Bessesen, D. H., C. L. Rupp, and R. H. Eckel. 1995. Dietary fat is shunted away from oxidation, toward storage in obese Zucker rats. *Obesity Research* 3:179–189.

Boozer, C. N., A. Brasseur, and R. L. Atkinson. 1993. Dietary fat affects weight loss and adiposity during energy restriction in rats. *American Journal of Clinical Nutrition* 58:846–852.

Boutelle, K. N., and D. S. Kirschenbaum. 1998. Further support for consistent self-monitoring as a vital component of successful weight control. *Obesity Research* 6:219–224.

Campbell, T. C., with T. M. Campbell. 2005. *The China Study: Startling implications for diet, weight loss, and long-term health*. Dallas: BenBella Books.

Ericsson, K. A., and N. Charness. 1994. Expert performance: Its structure and acquisition. *American Psychologist* 49:725–747.

Dobbing, J., ed. 1987. *Sweetness*. New York: Springer-Verlag.

Gately, P. J., C. B. Cooke, R. J. Butterly, P. Mackreth, and S. Carroll. 2000. The effects of a children's summer camp programme on weight loss, with a ten-month follow-up. *International Journal of Obesity* 24:1445–1453.

Geiselman, P. J., and D. Novin. 1982. The role of carbohydrates in appetite, hunger and obesity. *Appetite* 3:203–223.

Harris, J. K., S. A. French, R. W. Jeffery, P. McGovern, and R. R. Wing. 1994. Dietary and physical activity correlates of long-term weight loss. *Obesity Research* 2:307–313.

Hensen, C. J., L. C. Stevens, and J. R. Coast. 2001. Exercise duration and mood state: How much is enough to feel better? *Health Psychology* 20:267–275.

Hill, J. O., H. Drougas, and J. C. Peters. 1993. Obesity treatment: Can diet composition play a role? *Annals of Internal Medicine* 119:694–697.

How diet may protect against prostate cancer. *Tufts University Health & Nutrition Letter* 19:1,6.

Israel, A. C., and L. S. Shapiro. 1985. Behavior problems of obese children enrolling in a weight reduction program. *Cognitive Therapy and Research* 6:451–460.

Jeffery, R. W., W. L. Hellerstedt, S. A. French, and J. E. Baxter. 1995. A randomized trial of counseling for fat restriction versus calorie restriction in the treatment of obesity. *International Journal of Obesity* 19:132–137.

Kirschenbaum, D. S. 1987. Self-regulatory failure: A review with clinical implications. *Clinical Psychology Review* 7:77–104.

———. 1994. *Weight loss through persistence: Making science work for you.* Oakland, CA: New Harbinger.

———. 2000. *The nine truths about weight loss.* New York: Henry Holt.

———. 2006 *The healthy obsession program: Smart weight loss instead of low-carb lunacy.* Dallas: BenBella Books.

Kirschenbaum, D. S., R. D. Craig, K. P. Kelly, and J. N. Germann. 2007, under review. Immersion programs for the treatment of pediatric obesity: Two follow-up evaluations. Presented at the meetings of the North American Association for the Study of Obesity, 2005 and 2006.

———. 2007, under review. The first boarding school for overweight teenagers: Initial follow-up. Presented at the meeting of the North American Association for the Study of Obesity, 2005.

———. 2007, under review. Evaluation of two types of immersion programs for treating childhood and adolescent obesity: Academy of the Sierras (a therapeutic boarding school) and Wellspring Camps: *Obesity Management.*

Kirschenbaum, D. S., and P. Karoly. 1977. When self-regulation fails: Tests of some preliminary hypotheses. *Journal of Consulting and Clinical Psychology* 45:1116–1125.

McGuire, M. T., R. R. Wing, M. L. Klem, W. Lang, and J. O. Hill. 1999. What predicts weight regain in a group of successful weight losers? *Journal of Consulting and Clinical Psychology* 67:177–185.

———. 1999. Behavioral strategies of individuals who have maintained long-term weight losses. *Obesity Research* 7:334–341.

Perri, M. G., S. D. Anton, et al. 2002. Adherence to exercise prescriptions: Effects of prescribing moderate versus higher levels of intensity and frequency. *Health Psychology* 21:452–458.

Perri, M. G., A. M. Nezu, and B. J. Viegener. 1992. *Improving the long-term management of obesity: Theory, research and clinical guidelines.* New York: John Wiley.

Stice E. 1998. Prospective relation of dieting behaviors to weight change in a community sample of adolescents. *Behavior Therapy* 29:277–297.

Subrahmanyam, K., R. E. Kraut, P. M. Greenfield, and E. F. Gross. 2000. The impact of home computer use on children's activities and development. *Children and Computer Technology* 10:123–140.

Thayer, R. E. 1987. Energy, tiredness, and tension effects of a sugar snack versus moderate exercise. *Journal of Personality and Social Psychology* 52:119–125.

Wing, R. R., and J. O. Hill. 2001. Successful weight loss maintenance. *Annual Review of Nutrition* 21:323–341.

Index

Index

——

346